RECLAIMING THE URBAN COMMONS

About the editors

NICK ROSE is a specialist in the emerging fields of sustainable food systems, food sovereignty and food security. Nick received his PhD in Political Ecology from RMIT University for investigating the transformative potential of the global food sovereignty movement. He co-founded and coordinated the Australian Food Sovereignty Alliance (2010-2015), where he was one of the developers of Australia's first crowd-sourced food policy document, the People's Food Plan, jointly coordinated Fair Food Week, and was the Content Director of Australia's first food politics documentary, Fair Food. As Executive Director of Sustain: The Australian Food Network, he supports food system policy and programme work local government and beyond. Major initiatives include the Cardinia Food Circles project, the Melbourne Food Hub and the national Urban Agriculture Forum.

ANDREA GAYNOR is an Associate Professor of History at the University of Western Australia. An environmental historian, her research seeks to use the contextualising and narrative power of history to help solve real-world problems. Her doctoral research on the environmental history of food production in Australian cities was published by UWAP in 2006 as *Harvest of the Suburbs*. Her interests and expertise have subsequently expanded to encompass Western Australian environmental history, agricultural history, animals in history and the history of fish and fishing. She has undertaken research with diverse organisations including the Western Australian Department of Parks & Wildlife, Western Power and WWF-Australia, and among her forthcoming publications is a co-authored environmental history of Australia's southern mallee lands. She is currently researching histories of Landcare in Western Australia, water in Australian urbanisation and nature in Australian urban modernity, and teaching world environmental history and Australian history. At UWA she is Chair of the History Discipline Group and Director of the Centre for Western Australian History; she is also convenor of the Australian and New Zealand Environmental History Network and endeavours to influence policy as a member of The Beeliar Group: Professors for Environmental Responsibility.

RECLAIMING THE URBAN COMMONS

The past, present and future of food growing in Australian towns and cities

Edited by Nick Rose and Andrea Gaynor

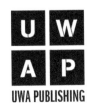
UWA PUBLISHING

First published in 2018 by
UWA Publishing
Crawley, Western Australia 6009
www.uwap.uwa.edu.au

UWAP is an imprint of UWA Publishing
a division of The University of Western Australia

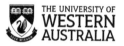

This book is copyright. Apart from any fair dealing for the purpose of private study, research, criticism or review, as permitted under the *Copyright Act 1968*, no part may be reproduced by any process without written permission. Enquiries should be made to the publisher.

Copyright © 2018

The moral right of the authors has been asserted.

All royalties from this work are being donated to Sustain: The Australian Food Network to further their work in supporting the transition to a healthy and sustainable Australian food system.

 A catalogue record for this book is available from the National Library of Australia

Cover design by Kate Pickard
Typeset in 11 point Bembo by Lasertype
Printed by Lightning Source

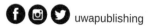 uwapublishing

This anthology is dedicated to the memory of Glenda Lindsay (1954–2017), gardener, singer, friend to many, active optimist, lover of the Earth and all her beings, organiser, connector, encourager, cook, delight to the eyes and the spirit and partner of Adrian.

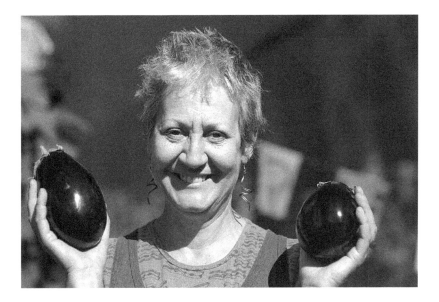

'Everything you do makes a difference for, whether you know it or not, other people gain confidence when you do something that you believe in.'
Glenda Lindsay

Urban agriculture is about people. Commoning is all about relationships. Glenda Lindsay, one of the guiding stars of urban agriculture in Melbourne, completely understood this. She connected people and inspired them to work together to make our everyday lives brighter and more beautiful. The planter boxes in Yarra streets and back lanes with their herbs, tomatoes and kale growing happily, cafes with plants on the pavement and guerrilla gardens, like

Tramstop 22, all exist thanks to her and the committees she helped establish. She shared her garden, Luscious Lane, led a Mexican Wave while singing at a Council meeting, created Compost Mates and a food swap. Numerous groups that are transforming our food system were started or supported by her.

She understood that inspiring people with gardening, food and song is the reweaving of connections between life, land, community and our inner selves. Her friendships went wide and deep, encompassing people from all over Australia as well as Africa and India. Wherever she went she gathered those who love the Earth and are working on healing. If you weren't like that when you met her, you certainly were soon after.

Glenda would be delighted with this book and all the hopeful and generous work it celebrates. No doubt she would appear, resplendent in mermaid earrings, dressed in fabric covered in fruits and vegetables, wearing a beanie in the shape of a strawberry and carrying a thermos flask of herbal tea and a plate of delicious mini-muffins to provide both celebration and enthusiastic support.

May this book spread confidence to many people to make steps they believe in to re-common us together in meaningful and restorative relationships.

Fran Murrell, Fitzroy, June 2018

Contents

Acknowledgements xi

Foreword: Recovering and Honouring Aboriginal Food
Systems in Twenty-first-century Australia xiii
Bruce Pascoe

Overview 1
Nick Rose and Andrea Gaynor

Introduction: Food as Urban Commons and
Community Economies 7
Katherine Gibson

Part 1: Many Australias
Chapter 1. Cultivating Stories in the Garden Across Cultures:
The R.A.W. Garden 17
Mariam Issa

Chapter 2. Preserving Calabrian Traditions in the Suburbs:
Rose Creek Estate, East Keilor 25
Gabriella Gomersall-Hubbard

CONTENTS

Chapter 3. Bringing Together Landless Farmers and Unused Farmland: The Sunraysia Burundian Garden and Food Next Door Initiative   39
Olivia Dun, Deborah Bogenhuber, Lesley Head, Joselyne Kadahari, Natascha Klocker, John Niyera and Joel Sindayigaya

Chapter 4. Cultivating Community   53
Peta Christensen

Part 2: Permaculture, Sustainability and Resilient Urban Food Systems

Chapter 5. Unearthing the Potential of Home Food Production   65
Kat Lavers and Hannah Moloney

Chapter 6. The Food Forest: Demonstrating a Sustainable Food Production System for Adelaide, South Australia   77
Graham and Annemarie Brookman

Chapter 7. Garden Farming: The Foundation for Agriculturally Productive Cities and Towns   91
David Holmgren

Chapter 8. Citizen Design, Permaculture and Community-based Urban Agriculture   101
Morag Gamble

Part 3: The New Face of Urban Agriculture in Australia

Chapter 9. Green World Revolution: Urban Farming as Social Enterprise   113
Toby Whittington and Ali Sumner

Chapter 10. The Wagtail Urban Farm Story   125
Steve Hoepfner

Chapter 11. Melbourne City Rooftop Honey 135
Vanessa Kwiatkowski and Mat Lumalasi

Chapter 12. Farming is Punk! 143
Joel Orchard

Chapter 13. Urban Food Street 155
Caroline Kemp

Part 4: Multiple Pasts, Possible Futures?
Chapter 14. Learning from our Productive Past 167
Andrea Gaynor

Chapter 15. Feeding Melbourne: Market Gardening in the Sandbelt, 1950s–1970s 175
Liz Clay

Chapter 16. Australia, 1945: The Future Begins 185
Srebrenka Kunek and John Shone

Conclusion: Laying the Foundations for Sustainable Urban Food Systems in Australia 197
Nick Rose

Appendix: The Urban Agriculture Manifesto 205

Notes 211

Acknowledgements

We are extremely grateful to all the authors of the various chapters and their collaborators. Everyone gave generously of their time and replied conscientiously and with good humour and grace to our many requests as editors. We would also like to thank all those who kindly provided images, and Philip Webster for his cheerful and efficient assistance with formatting the final manuscript.

We are also very grateful to University of Western Australia Publishing for their commitment to this project and their hard work in turning the manuscript into a book. The support and encouragement of UWAP Director Terri-ann White and Publishing Manager Kate Pickard have been invaluable, as has the careful editing performed by Melanie Dankel.

Nick Rose and Andrea Gaynor, Melbourne/Perth, July 2018

Foreword

Recovering and Honouring Aboriginal Food Systems in Twenty-first-century Australia

Bruce Pascoe

Australia is a colonised country with a colonial mind. The first Europeans were steadfast in their refusal to use the food offered by this country, the domesticated food products of Aboriginal Australians. It was a point of colonial pride not to go native, not to have anything to do with the products of Australia. Thus, we stuck to suet pudding, potatoes, mutton, grapes, wheat, barley and so on. We hungered for the English homeland and insisted on eating roast beef and Yorkshire pudding on Christmas day, mutton and peas, pork with apple sauce. All of those foods require nutrients and moisture levels that Australia cannot provide, so we introduced superphosphate from the phosphate barons of the Pacific Islands; we plundered the waters of this dry continent, seemingly intent on destroying those finite reserves. Rivers where early settlers barged cheese and milk and vegetables hundreds of kilometres inland are no longer navigable by canoe, such is our mistreatment of those sacred waters. Applying English ploughing techniques to the light and friable Australian soils has caused metres of topsoil to blow into the rivers and seas. We've abused this continent because of our refusal to fully understand the land's needs. Now is the time for us to look carefully at this continent, turn respectfully to Mother Earth, apologise for our abuse and consider how we might live within the means of our soil and climate and treat Australia as if it were itself and not somewhere else. Let's grow Australian plants and develop a truly Australian cuisine. And not just the condiments of mountain pepper and bush tomato, but the staples as well, the grains and tubers, most of which are perennial and drought tolerant and thus kind to the soil and less demanding of our precious water. Our environment will thank us and so will our tastebuds and bellies.

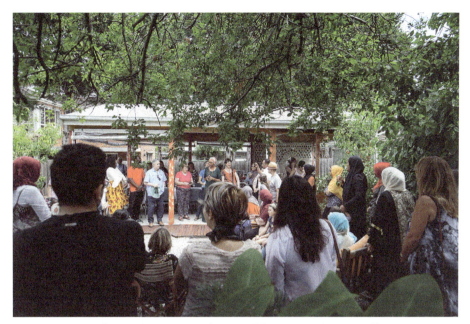

Figure 1.3. Storytelling at the RAW Garden in collaboration with Story Tellers Victoria. Photo courtesy of Tatiana Scott.

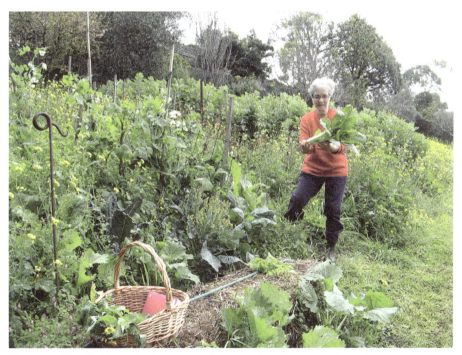

Figure 2.5. Lina Siciliano picking the evening meal from the vegetable garden. Photo courtesy of Gabriella Gomersall-Hubbard.

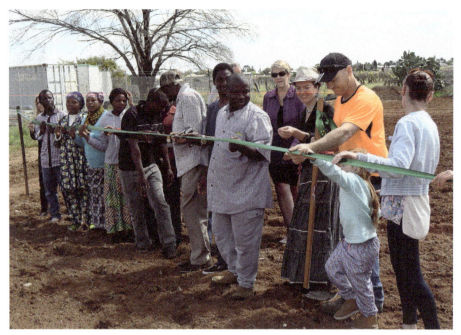

Figure 3.3. Cutting the ribbon at the official opening ceremony of the Sunraysia Burundian Garden. Photo courtesy of Olivia Dun.

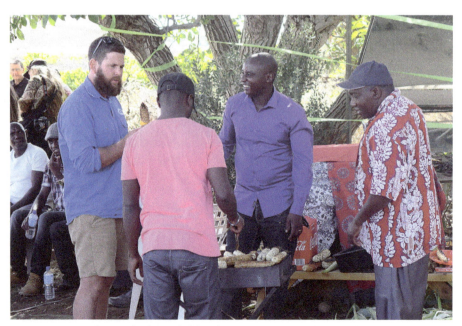

Figure 3.6. Maize harvest barbecue held at the Sunraysia Burundian Garden in February 2017. Photo courtesy of Olivia Dun.

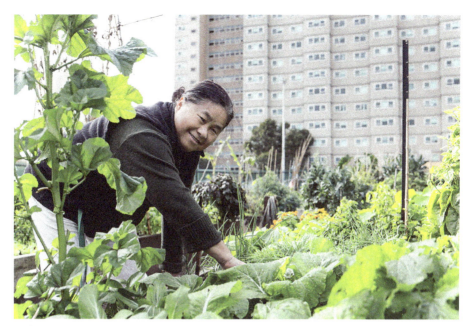

Figure 4.1. Kim Chua tends her bountiful plot of leafy greens and herbs in the Collingwood Public Housing Estate Community Garden. Photo courtesy of Greg Elms.

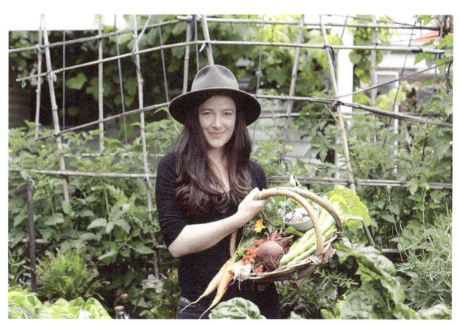

Figure 5.3. Kat Lavers in the kitchen garden at the Plummery. Photo courtesy of Amy Piesse Photography.

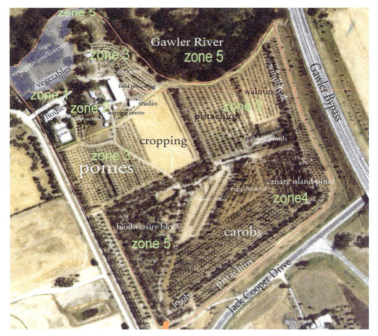

Figure 6.1. Aerial image of the Food Forest, Adelaide, with permaculture zones marked. Photo courtesy of Graham Brookman.

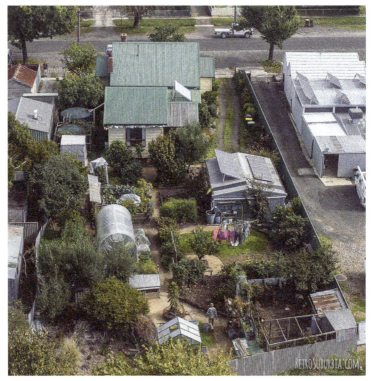

Figure 7.1. Garden farming in Australian suburbs. Photo courtesy of Holmgren Design.

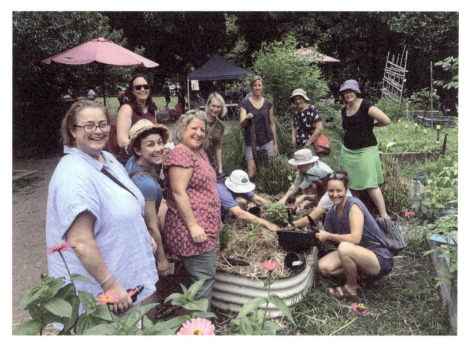

Figure 8.3. Even established projects like Northey Street City Farm have places where new groups can add richness and detail. This group designed and planted a tea garden near the community kitchen. Photo courtesy of Morag Gamble.

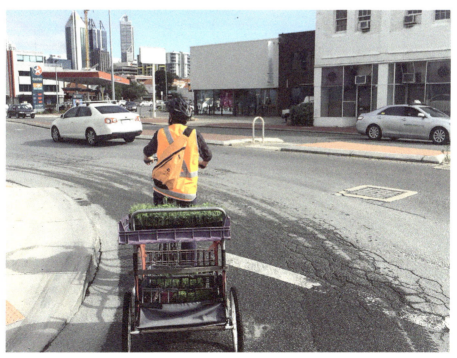

Figure 9.2. Craig, unemployed for four years prior to getting a job with Green World Revolution, delivering Gladstone Street Urban Farm produce into the Perth CBD, spring 2016. Photo courtesy of Toby Whittington and Ali Sumner.

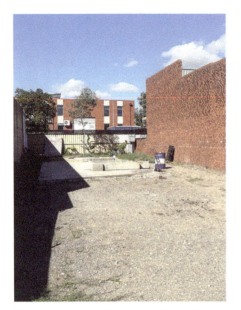
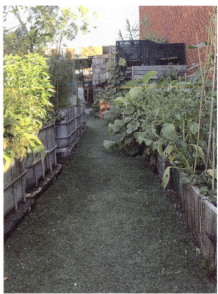

Figures 9.3a and b. The site of Green World Revolution's first urban farm, the Gladstone Street Farm in East Perth, in winter 2013 (L) and summer 2016 (R). Photos courtesy of Toby Whittington and Ali Sumner.

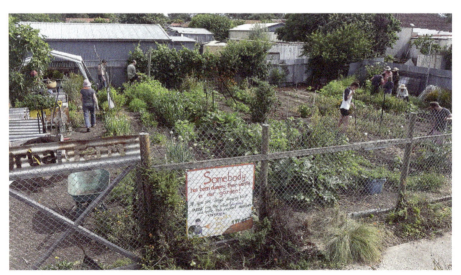

Figure 10.4. A working bee at Wagtail Farm involving trellising, weeding, a mega composting session and generally preparing the site for summer planting. Photo courtesy of Steven Hoepfner.

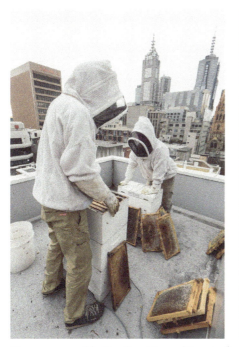
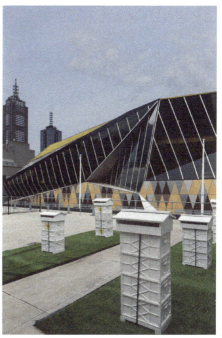

Figure 11.1a and b. Rooftop Honey hives in the Melbourne CBD: Degraves Street and the Emporium. Photo courtesy of Anneliese Henjak.

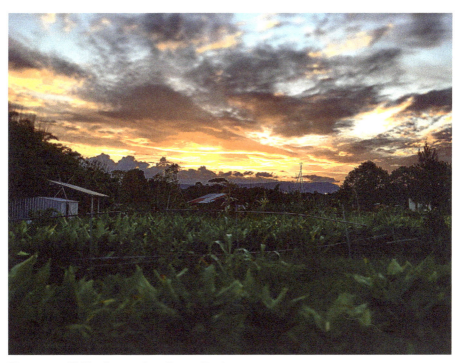

Figure 12.1. Fields of turmeric at Future Feeders. Photo courtesy of Joel Orchard.

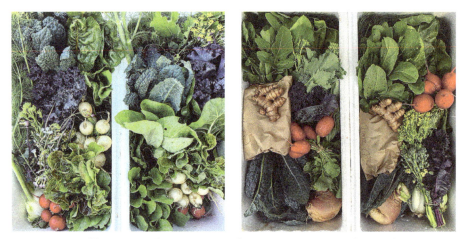

Figure 12.3 a and b. Spring and autumn seasonal Community Supported Agriculture (CSA) vegie boxes. Photo courtesy of Joel Orchard.

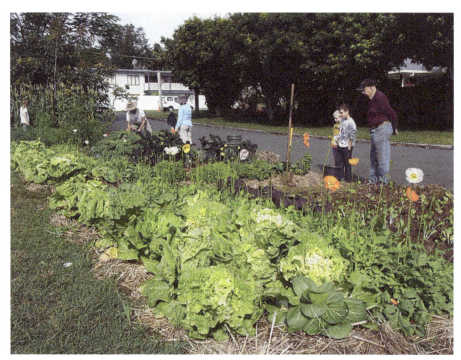

Figure 13.2. This photo was taken at the end of a working bee in the Market Garden (Farnwyn Court). This garden was removed voluntarily by the home owner once the council demanded permits and insurance. It produced 2,400 units of winter greens (bok choy, pak choy, kale, lettuce) in a three-month period over winter, demonstrating how productive these spaces can be. Photo courtesy of Caroline Kemp.

Overview

Nick Rose and Andrea Gaynor

When we first proposed this anthology, *Reclaiming the Urban Commons: The past, present and future of food growing in Australian towns and cities,* we did so with a number of aims in mind. First, building on the legacy of Andrea's ground-breaking research published as *Harvest of the Suburbs* in 2006, we wanted to continue the ongoing work of uncovering and revealing little-known or long-forgotten histories of urban and peri-urban food production in Australia. Secondly, we wanted to provide space for some of the country's leading innovators and practitioners of urban agriculture to share their stories of what they are doing, how they are doing it and why. And thirdly, by synthesising leading case studies and lessons of the past and present of urban food growing in Australia, we wanted to stimulate what we and many others believe are necessary reflections on our current predicament. These reflections are not an idle intellectual exercise. On the contrary, they are an attempt to grapple with matters that go to the heart of how – and whether – we continue to inhabit this land in the coming decades of this century and beyond.

As all the contributors to this anthology explicitly or implicitly recognise, we are in the midst of a great shift, a fundamental transformation in our relations with the Earth and with each other. This shift has many dimensions, however, it fundamentally poses humanity with this challenge, to paraphrase Thomas Berry:

> *How can humanity transition from a period of devastation of the Earth and its multitude of lifeforms – including ourselves – to a period when we can be present to the planet in a mutually beneficial manner?*[1]

What we believe this collection shows is that the response to that existential and evolutionary question must be grounded in a transformed relationship to the land and to each other. As argued by Bruce Pascoe in the foreword, and as demonstrated by the stories narrated in these pages, this transformation begins with a deeper knowledge of and connection to our food. Such knowledge, when translated into daily practices and ways of being and inhabiting this country, has the potential to ultimately bring about the paradigm shift required to live well in this place and to live at peace with ourselves and one another.

At a time of increasing fear, division and xenophobia, the urgent and too-long-delayed task of truth-telling, recovery of historical memory, healing and reconciliation between Aboriginal and non-Aboriginal Australians can provide a beacon of hope towards the future. The path lit by that beacon shows life-sustaining practices of care, respect and responsibility to the land, as well as delight in the diverse array of delicious produce that it bestows upon us.

This is the future that is already emerging, glimpses of which are captured in the stories that follow in these pages. A few years ago, humanity passed the critical tipping point of becoming for the first time a truly urban species. Australia is grappling with a trajectory of increasing urbanisation in what is already one of the world's most urbanised countries. The question of how to design, build and live well in our cities and towns has never been more critical. To this we must add that the country's major public health challenges are now explicitly linked to poor diet, and the dynamic of seemingly endless urban sprawl coupled with the loss of farmer viability poses a direct and serious challenge to current and future food security in a context of global political instability and non-linear climate change. Therefore, the challenge of how we both *live and eat well* in our urbanised present and near future is one that demands our urgent attention and prioritisation.

This is the challenge that all the contributors to this anthology have addressed. Following on from the vital and succinct reminder and injunction from Bruce Pascoe, Professor Katherine Gibson sets the scene in her introductory chapter, which explores the meaning and practices of *commoning* and in particular the idea of food as an urban commons. As she suggests, *commoning* is best understood as a verb, embodying a constellation of practices reflective of particular values and social relations. It is these practices and values that are then articulated in the following chapters.

Part 1 contains four chapters, each of which reflects the wealth of diversity that exists in current practices of urban and peri-urban edible gardening and agriculture in a selection of locations in Melbourne and Victoria. In chapter 1, Somali-born author and speaker Mariam Issa shares her story of building R.A.W. (Resilient Aspiring Women), a community of women in Melbourne's southern suburbs, offering the profound insight that our strength comes from acknowledging the vulnerability within all of us once we recognise our fundamental interdependence and interconnection. Gabriella Gomersall-Hubbard (chapter 2) narrates Lina and Tony Siciliano's wonderful three-decade (re-)creation of a little piece of Calabria in East Keilor, replete with olive groves, vineyards, heritage chickens and a flourishing market garden. Olivia Dun and her co-authors in chapter 3 describe the uplifting collaboration that has seen local food community advocates in Mildura work with members of the Burundian community to transform small vacant urban plots into the inspiring Food Next Door project, which has created access to healthy and culturally important food as well as much-needed livelihood opportunities. Finally, in chapter 4, Peta Christensen shares the moving story of Cultivating Community: how the cultural needs and demands of diverse migrant communities living in social housing in inner-Melbourne municipalities were met by the creation of dozens of allotment gardens, with the support of the Victorian Office of Housing.

Part 2 acknowledges the critically important role played by the permaculture movement in training and inspiring a whole generation of urban and peri-urban gardeners and farmers. It begins with two leading members of the vanguard of this movement, Kat Lavers and Hannah Moloney, reflecting in chapter 5 on their experiences of creating and sustaining themselves and others from bountiful home gardens in Melbourne and Hobart respectively. In chapter 6, Graham and Annemarie Brookman recount their three-decade journey of adaptive ecological learning, design and resilience in the world-renowned Food Forest at Gawler, north of Adelaide. David Holmgren, co-originator of the permaculture movement back in the mid-1970s, reflects on the cycles of interest in what he terms 'garden farming' and the 'home-based non-monetary economy' in chapter 7, with a focus on the latest and potentially most transformative cycle, which David has captured in his important new book, *RetroSuburbia*. This part concludes in chapter 8 with the story of one of Queensland's leading exponents of permaculture, Morag Gamble, reflecting on the early days of the iconic Northey Street City Farm, embodying the principles and practices of what she terms 'citizen designers'.

Part 3 contains five chapters on what we have termed 'the new face of urban agriculture in Australia'. These five stories are expressions of the diversity of experimentation underway across the country, each demonstrating elements of what we regard as the core characteristics of *urban commoning*:

- sharing and collaboration,
- connection and interdependence,
- nurturing, care, respect and trust,
- celebration, joy, welcoming and hospitality,
- healing and overcoming,
- creativity, and
- diversity.

In chapter 9, Toby Whittington and Ali Sumner share their story of the creation of the Perth-based social enterprise Green World Revolution – to date, one of the very few economically viable urban farming and social enterprise operations in Australia. Steve Hoepfner (chapter 10) speaks of the friendship, camaraderie, hard work and passion that led to the flourishing of Wagtail Urban Farm in Adelaide. In chapter 11 we read about how one couple, Vanessa Kwiatkowski and Mat Lumalasi, decided to take action on the global issue of the dwindling number of honeybees and, in the process, created a successful urban agriculture social enterprise, Melbourne Rooftop Honey. Young Mullumbimby-based urban farmer Joel Orchard (chapter 12) shares his journey into farming as the best means by which he could express his deep environmental activism and his desire to reconnect with the earth, leading to the formation of the Future Feeders collective and with the promise of a Young Farmers Network for Australia. In chapter 13, Caroline Kemp narrates the inspiring, but also salutary, story of the re-imaging of a hitherto bland suburban streetscape in Buderim, Sunshine Coast, into a dynamic neighbourhood connected through a network of edible trees and verge plants, which she and her partner Duncan McNaught dubbed 'Urban Food Street'.

In Part 4, three chapters reflect on the past and present of urban and peri-urban agriculture in Australia. In a brief reprise of *Harvest of the Suburbs*, Andrea Gaynor (chapter 14) notes the long trajectory and desire of urban populations in Australia for diverse ways to achieve food self-provisioning, highlighting the significance of class and gender amid changing access to land, time and legal capacity for food production from the nineteenth to twenty-first centuries. Liz Clay (chapter 15) provides a highly personal reflection on her childhood growing up on a 60-acre family market garden in Keysborough in Melbourne's sandbelt to the southeast. It was the market gardens of the sandbelt that satisfied the growing city's demand for fruit and vegetables for 100 years, largely coming to an end in the 1970s with the rewards of housing subdivision winning out over the need for horticulture close to the city. Finally, in chapter 16, Srebrenka Kunek and John Shone link this dynamic of sprawl and the consequent devaluing of farming and farmland to the very conscious shift in economic development and, specifically, migration policy in the post–World War II decades, with a particular focus on the southern European immigration program.

In the concluding chapter, Nick Rose brings these narrative strands together, re-stating the case for the urgency of transformative practice and policy as well as the central role that urban agriculture in all its diverse forms must play in the articulation of the emerging story of the sustainable and flourishing future for Australia that we believe will be written as this century draws to a close.

Introduction

Food as Urban Commons and Community Economies

Katherine Gibson

'A community makes and shares a commons…Without a commons, there is no community, without a community, there is no commons.'

Stephen Gudeman[1]

'Urban commoning is the messy, everyday, necessarily compromised work of trying to build networks of survival in the midst of the high-pressure centrality of the urban.'

Amanda Huron[2]

A 'commons' is a property, practice or knowledge that is shared by a community and that contributes to community survival and well-being. As the opening quotes illustrate, there has been a shift in framing, from thinking about the commons as a thing, a noun, to *commoning* as a verb, as something that is done. This shift, prompted by the foundational work of Peter Linebaugh,[3] is being made by many people today who are interested in making other possible worlds. What Stephen Gudeman highlights, however, is that a community is necessary to a commons and is constituted in the act of commoning.

But the making of a commoning community – including its rules about access, use, responsibility, benefit and ownership, its bounded inclusions and inevitable exclusions – is, as Amanda Huron points out, a messy and experimental business. This is especially so in the urban context where privatised property relations dominate and where monetised exchange prevails over practices of subsistence. So, what does it mean to talk of food as an urban commons? In this introductory essay, I explore this question through stories about food production in urban settings, starting with my own experience of growing up in Sydney in a diverse food economy that became increasingly homogeneous and moving on to stories that illustrate the growing interest in food commoning in urban settings.

Theories and conceptual categories are performative of the world we inhabit – they make some things more real and place other things in the shadows. *Reclaiming the Urban Commons: The past, present and future of food growing in Australian towns and cities* is shedding light on a whole range of urban agricultural practices that have been largely overlooked in the histories of Australian urbanisation. The urban has been set apart from the rural, where food growing 'rightly' seemed to belong. But, as I hope to illustrate, food provisioning and practices of commoning have always been entwined in the entanglements of urban and rural life. Today, more than half of the world's population lives in cities and there is much interest in 'taking back' the food economy both in rural areas and in cities so that it contributes directly to the health of people and the planet.[4] It is important see food production as a contested site of both commoning *and* uncommoning, community making *and* unmaking, so that we can take steps to build ethically oriented community economies that make the benefits of an urban food commons more real.

As a child of the 1950s who was raised in suburban Sydney, my memories of food growing are many and varied. For years these memories have lain unexamined, seemingly unremarkable until now, when I look back and attempt a retrospective inventory of the diverse economy of food production that existed around me as I grew up and the way that commoning and uncommoning was performed. I remember our chook house and its inhabitants located at the end of the backyard next to the swing my father had built. It was a raised platform with a roof and wire sides. When our feathered egg producers were sacked sometime around the beginning of the 1960s, the chook house became a proxy stage, albeit one facing a fence, on which I enjoyed a brief performing career – before it was taken down to be replaced by a 'landscaped' garden. This rather alluring image referred to the replacement of straight lines in the garden with curvy edges and tiered plantings. The chooks and their house had no place in such an arty, upwardly mobile environment where the garden was no longer a site of food production but one of display and distinction. Fresh home-grown eggs gave way to shop-bought ones; a market transaction replaced self-provisioning. The more-than-human community of human and chicken commoners who had once made and shared a garden home was no more – it had been 'uncommoned'.

In my memory, growing vegetables continued in most of the backyards I visited for play purposes during the 1950s. At one friend's place, we would be paid a penny per bucket of snails that we collected from the choko vine. The grandparents' backyards were especially productive, with fruit trees as well as chooks and vegetable patches. The ability to grow food had been crucial during the war years of food scarcity, and the habits of self-provisioning were hard to give up. The skills and know-how to grow food was a tacit knowledge that circulated around the neighbourhood and between generations in families. So, while growing and harvesting took place in the privacy of the family backyard, there was a shared open-access knowledge commons that supported urban food production. The community that maintained and passed on this knowledge commons was made up of men and women who had come through the war, coped with rationing and had access to (though not necessarily ownership of) plots of suburban land. They shared a set of tastes probably originating in their Anglo-Irish heritage: potatoes, pumpkins, peas, beans, carrots and silverbeet were the preferred crops. This was an era before broccoli, zucchini, garlic and herbs were commonplace.

At this time, the connections between urban and rural Australia were more immediate. Many families had relatives on the land or in rural centres and the movement of food into cities was not only via commercial transactions. Relatives would send boxes of home-grown produce on the train down to the city where family members would pick up the bottled fruit, side of lamb, fresh vegetables and baked goods that could be shared. Children were packed off to relatives over the holidays and got to experience aspects of rural life, including seeing where food came from. As a primary school student, I went on a week-long excursion to the Murrumbidgee Irrigation Area (MIA) and Snowy Mountains Scheme where we were billeted with families of primary school children all over southern NSW, including on an orange-growing farm in the MIA and, much to my delight, with a family who owned and lived above a milk bar in Cooma. Unremarkable as it then was to me, I experienced a diverse economy of food production involving self-provisioning, small business, smallholder intensive farming and more extensive family farming.

The post-war economic boom saw industrialised agriculture and manufacturing factory production take over many areas of the food system resulting in the production of cheaper food that was marketed to consumers by an increasingly sophisticated advertising industry. By the mid- to late 1960s, backyard veggie patches seemed to have gone the way of homemade Carnation Milk ice cream – banished to another age. Food packages from the rural hinterlands were an anomaly. The food knowledge commons that had once been actively cared for and maintained by urban and rural communities alike contracted and became fragmented. Now practices of self-provisioning appeared to be a remarkable, even undesirable outlier – especially when it involved 'new Australians' growing unfamiliar things like eggplant, olives and artichokes in front yards, transgressing the neat suburban display aesthetic. The urban food-knowledge commons went underground and became the 'property' of certain migrant communities.

As the Great Acceleration of economic growth and associated environmental degradation took off,[5] I witnessed urban development spreading out to cover food-producing land with concrete and asphalt. The rural-urban fringe surrounding Sydney was still relatively close in during the 1980s when I took university geography students on field trips to the Hills district to see family-owned and -run dairy farms and market gardens. Today, this area is the province of dual-income commuter households in two-storey houses occupying almost the whole block, bar the paved driveway. The suburban garden has been reduced to a narrow strip of grass or astro-turf and a few strategically placed, low-maintenance ornamental plants. In such an environment, self-provisioning and urban agriculture is largely impossible. Where it persists, such as around Richmond on the fertile soils of the Nepean River flats, urban residents are up in arms about chemical pollution or unpleasant odours and co-existence is threatened.

It is tempting to read the history of food production during the Great Acceleration in Australia as a history of *uncommoning*. Communities have experienced the loss of shared knowledge about food-growing practices and there has been reduced access to food-producing land in cities. Individuated as isolated consumers, community members have seen responsibility for food growing handed over to the industrial food system and provisioning to centralised retailers. The economic benefits of food-production flow to multinational, profit-oriented companies and the nutritional benefits flowing to the consumer are increasingly under question.

Yet, it is in this context that we have seen a remarkable rise of interest in taking back the food economy so that it contributes directly to the health of people and the planet. A reinstated language of the commons and commoning has been central to this movement. In our densifying cities, people have come together to reclaim land for urban gardening. At perhaps the smallest scale, kerbsides have been commoned for food production and flower growing. Here, the community of commoners is made up of householders who live on certain streets, walkers along those streets and animals and insects who frequent the streets or are attracted to the gardens and the vegetation itself. *Access* to the kerbside commons is public; the forms of *use* are usually negotiated with local councils who formally 'own' the roads, pavements and verges; self-designated gardeners take *responsibility* for the *maintenance* and *care* of the verge gardens and members of the general public and animals and insects *benefit* from the output, be it pleasurable visuals, aromas, touch sensations or edible produce. The boundaries of the commoning community are loosely defined but are relatively local. The durability of the verge food commons is dependent on the negotiating skill of all the members of this multi-species community. Contestation and experimentation are the constant accompaniments of commoning.[6]

At a larger scale, we have seen privately and publicly owned land converted into community gardens that have become an urban commons. In Newcastle, NSW, for example, pocket parks, unused bowling greens and vacant blocks have been commoned by groups of people who have organised *access* to sites, established rules of *use*, taken *responsibility* for managing the site, *maintained* the gardens and other activities and shared the *benefit* of food produce and environmental amenity to a wider community.[7] This commoning of land has been accompanied by the commoning of knowledge about urban food production in the local context. Many of those communities who had maintained culturally grounded food commons knowledge are now celebrated as major contributors to the multicultural food landscape. And this landscape has become even more complex as new arrivals to Australia bring growing skills and new food preferences that are showcased at urban farms such as the Mamre House in Sydney's west.[8]

In the process of getting hands dirty in the raised beds and garden plots of community gardens, there is a sharing of wider knowledge about the food system. Surplus community garden output is regularly donated to community feeding programs, such as OzHarvest, which redirects food to target groups experiencing food insecurity and keeps food waste out of landfill. Such networks of alternative food provisioning constitute another community of volunteer commoners whose efforts are focused on people-to-people distributional strategies that bypass the market or reclaim value from market discards.

As food commoning has become more visible in urban settings, we have seen the radical diversification of the food economy. The homogeneous industrial food landscape that began to emerge in Australia during the 1960s has been squarely challenged by the development of niche markets for organic produce; heritage strains of grains, fruits and vegetables; local farmers markets; fair-trade networks; and the resurgence and celebration of home production. Chooks are back and possibly even choko vines!

What we are seeing across a broad front are the elements of a community food economy coming into being. A community (as opposed to a capitalist) economy foregrounds being-in-common and our necessary interdependence with each other and earth others.[9] Its analytics focus upon ethical negotiations around:

- the diverse labours involved in surviving well socially and ecologically,

- encounters with producers and environments both near and far,
- surplus production, appropriation and distribution,
- commoning the property, practices and knowledge that support life and
- investing in futures so that future generations can live well.

Food is central to living well and its production for human subsistence is our primary way of interacting with the earth others who sustain us. In urban areas, we are witnessing an awakening to the role that food plays in building healthy communities. Practices of urban food commoning have come out of the shadows and are signalling one way forward to other possible worlds.

PART 1

Many Australias

Chapter 1

Cultivating Stories in the Garden Across Cultures: The R.A.W. Garden

Mariam Issa

The R.A.W (Resilient Aspiring Women) Garden sprouted from a premise my mother always shared with us: 'If you can host one in your heart, you can host them in your home'. Growing up, I could not fathom the meaning of these words and their weight eluded me for quite a while. Now, however, having operated the R.A.W. Garden for six years, I am finally starting to capture the significance of her words.

When our habits are born of honest intentions, they become our rituals and traditions, and in time these become the values by which our lives are governed. These values can be shared across cultures and nations, and they can become the bridge that connects us at a deeper level because of our shared memories.

When we share commonality in traditions, we share commonality in values: what I would define as our cultural currency. A currency that can remind us of the happy shared memories – an anchor that holds and connects us in deep and meaningful ways in times of upheavals and breakdowns.

When my family and I came to Australia as refugees, our cultural currency was unknown; no one knew or shared our traditions. Our

predicament was that we had come from a shared communal culture where:
- well-being was attained through loyalty to the collective,
- independent thinking was not common, and
- identity was not individual but shared with the whole.

In this strange new world, we faced a constant battle with our inner selves. It was far from the utopian world we imagined and we were forced to re-create ourselves in relation to the new community. Why? Because none of our traditions were practiced in the same way and we were not sure if our values aligned. A decade after our arrival and having acquired a levelled comprehension of the community we now called home, a few seemingly simple, yet complex issues became apparent to us.

Firstly, in our different traditions, there were things we shared and had in common, and, in fact, our *shared values* seemed to be more than our *differences*. Secondly, *trust* was a key element in living and accepting each other's values. Thirdly, *fear*, we realised, was one of the factors that was impeding our living harmoniously together.

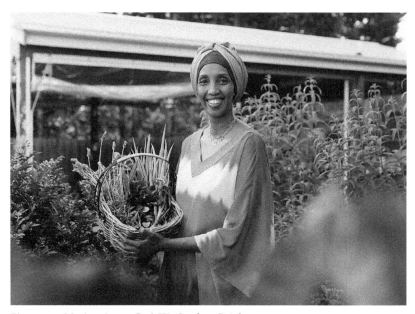

Figure 1.1. Mariam Issa at R.A.W. Garden, Brighton. Photo courtesy of Tatiana Scott.

Having recognised not only the presence but also the reality of these huge gaps, I took it upon myself to address this malady. How so? By accepting it as my integration assignment. In pursuing it I found some key insights:
- no one is ever put somewhere randomly, and
- there are forces beyond us and our comprehension that always draw us together to remind each other of what we've forgotten of ourselves.

I cannot say it was an easy journey for myself or my family, but we somehow discovered the values we'd forgotten in our new community and we made it our duty to remind it of the values they'd forgotten about themselves.

In our African oral traditions, it is said, 'It takes a whole village to raise a child,' and I, coming from these traditions, add, 'When we nurture the woman, we nurture the village.' This is the seed from which my passion for connecting women and creating a safe environment for the community sprouted.

R.A.W. is an incorporated, not-for-profit organisation and it operates as a community garden in my backyard. My inspiration for R.A.W. comes from my love and passion for working with women and the community after my journey as a refugee to a proud woman who belongs in the Melbourne community. I derived a wealth of knowledge and life skills from the community that embraced me when I was a refugee, and I want to reciprocate the favour and share the wealth and wisdom of my East African traditions and heritage with the fast-paced urban community in which I now live.

Our aim for R.A.W. was to close the inter-generational gap and bring women of all ages, diverse cultural backgrounds and abilities together to experience the joy of community. We wanted women and like-minded individuals to come together and have a space for cultural exchange and shared stories, to be able to participate in social events and take part in productive workshops amongst other fulfilling activities. We issued an invitation to the community to remember the simple joys of gardening and the benefit it provides to our health and our environment. Finally, we wanted to share our diversity by creating spaces for interaction between migrants, refugees and mainstream Australians.

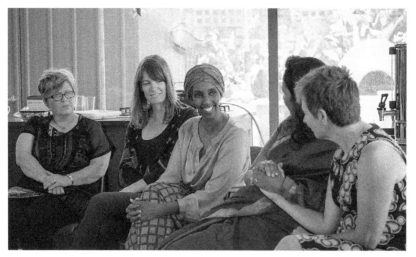

Figure 1.2. Storytelling at the R.A.W. Garden in collaboration with Story Tellers Victoria. Photo courtesy of Tatiana Scott.

Some memories that I reminisce on quite fondly include how my grandmother used to host circles of women in our home when she visited us – these circles are a Somali tradition where women come together for '*shah* and *sheko*', which simply translates as 'tea and stories'. This was a safe space for women to connect deeply and to be brave enough to be vulnerable with one another. It was usually a Friday afternoon ritual and it had a sort of ceremonial aspect to it, where my grandmother deep-fried coffee beans in corn oil and made popcorn. The popcorn was then eaten with dates. Coffee oil was used for healing purposes: I believe it was mainly to ease the body's stresses (the oil was also used for massages for expectant mothers or for babies before their bath).

I believe this simple act of women coming together served many purposes. It was a safe space to share their turmoil and their happiness at the same time. The coffee roasted in oil and its by-products not only provided an aromatic fragrance but infused the feeling of safety, reassurance, support and unity. Rituals like dance and composing poetry were part of it, and I also remember it was a space where marriages were initiated. Women were the ones who knew the best match for their sons and daughters and this was the place for matchmaking.

A couple of months before I incorporated the R.A.W. organisation, I was struggling with what to name it. One night, however, I had a dream and the name R.A.W. was presented to me. I remember the precise time I woke up (2 am) and I wrote the name R.A.W. on a piece of paper and went back to sleep. Unbeknownst to me, R.A.W. translated to Resilient Aspiring Women – someone once told me that R.A.W. backwards reads WAR! This was a perfect metaphor for my life and captured the very essence of what I was about to bring in whatever capacity I could: mentally, emotionally and spiritually.

I had harboured a lot of war in the turbulent waters of my heart and I knew that only when I could gather the courage to self-examine my inner world would I still those waters and be reminded of my resilience and aspirations for life again.

R.A.W. also meant going back to the simplicity of life and sharing our stories, such as the one I touched on about my grandmother's rituals. And it also meant going back to the foundations of respecting and connecting with Mother Earth. I believe deeply that each and every woman, like me, has those turbulent waters that need calming and she harbours a war inside that she needs to let go of. A big part of R.A.W. is inspiring women to not only stop these wars, but also win them! Well, the best place I know to do this is in a garden. Why? Mother Earth is ready to support us in our traditions of healing, and when we do this, her reciprocated action heals us back.

I incorporated the organisation as not for profit and found not only incredible, but also formidable women who supported me through the journey. We laid our foundation with intention, that intent being: 'All women who will benefit the garden and will benefit from it will come on their own'. R.A.W. would operate fully autonomously where *trust* was the key for its *growth*. We invited the community to adopt a tree and then we asked them to create an intention for their tree, to identify what was missing in their world and what they wanted to bring alive in this space. We had a tree-planting day and when my mother-in-law was given the opportunity to plant her tree, she said, 'I want my tree to be one of abundance'. That same year her apple tree had the most sweet and abundant fruit. Intentions are powerful and they do come to fruition.

There are myriad issues that need addressing in communities, such as isolation, ostracism, emotional health, mental health and physical health, amongst others. In order to address these issues as a community in our urban world, we need community gardens and spaces where people can feel safe to share their stories. R.A.W. has shown us how a simple initiative like ours can have a powerful impact in our diverse community. These spaces also have the power to welcome marginalised community members who might be going through vulnerable times.

From simple conversations and random acts of kindness, we now have a thriving organic garden and an orchard with more than thirty fruitful trees. One of our greatest hurdles early on was earning the trust of the community. However, with the resilience and aspirations of our volunteer spirit, we earned the trust of community members and that of people in positions of influence. A pavilion to carry out our activities was built for us by Rotarians and another philanthropic organisation built us a top-notch kitchen, while a church community designed and built our paths. The garden now opens every Tuesday and Sunday. People from around the community come to the garden, share stories, create arts and crafts and through cooking classes partake in the wealth of cuisine from the different and diverse countries we all come from; we've had more than twelve different cuisines from various nations. We partner and collaborate with great organisations like

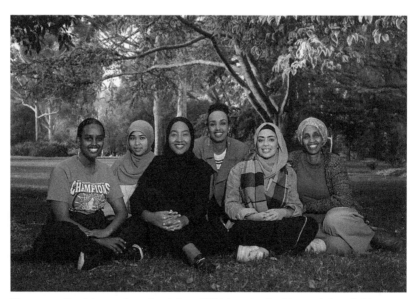

Figure 1.4. Participants from Lead from Within, a leadership workshop led by Mariam Issa. Photo courtesy of Tatiana Scott.

Storytellers Victoria, Igniting Change (a philanthropic organisation passionate about supporting local and diverse communities), Scanlon Foundation (which is passionate about social cohesion), Rotary (working to close the gaps for community), Victorian Multicultural Commission, Bayside City Council and many local community organisations, especially the Castlefield community centre.

As a gardener, I understand the seed of potential inherent in all of us, and in this journey I am reporting back from experience that community exists, and that when we put aside our fears and ignorance, we've a great adventure ahead of us – a thrilling adventure through which we can plant the seeds of many beautiful forests with great intentions. When we share our simple, joyful stories, we can grow a healthy and resilient community where people are happy and joyful; this is how we can thrive together and lift the veil of ignorance and intolerance in us.

Both our individual and collective worlds are in transition and humanity is going through the remembrance of our true ideal: creating a sustainable world for each other. We cannot continue in ignorance and I believe the call is subconsciously coming from us as

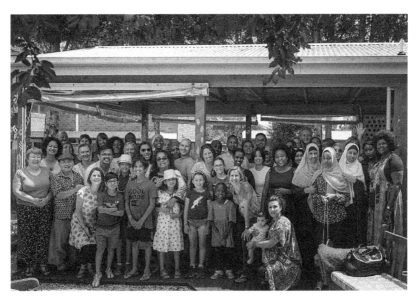

Figure 1.5. Welcome Lunch in collaboration with R.A.W.'s sister organisation Space2b. Photo courtesy of Tatiana Scott.

a collective to be a support for each other. In the simple community garden in my backyard I've learned to be vulnerable with others, and through this I have come to the realisation that our vulnerability is our biggest strength – we're not self-made, we are interconnected and interdependent and the more we remember and understand this, the better chance we have for a smooth transformation. My family and I have also learned a great lesson in acceptance and, since opening our backyard and hosting people in our home, we've been reminded that family exists beyond blood relations. I don't see any better way to do this than to connect more with our common values and our shared humanity, for our world is demanding it.

The R.A.W. Garden is now a great platform where inspired women convene, where we practice the affirmation that dreams can be realised effortlessly through our shared synergy. This ties well with my mother's simple saying, 'if we can host someone in our hearts, we can host them in our homes'. I believe my mother's legacy lives in me and hopefully it will be shared through many more generations to come!

Chapter 2

Preserving Calabrian Traditions in the Suburbs: Rose Creek Estate, East Keilor

Gabriella Gomersall-Hubbard

Only 20 kilometres from Melbourne's city centre, Rose Creek Estate is probably one of the most urban farms in Australia and one of the most intriguing. The casual passer-by would never think that behind the red-brick facade of one of the houses in suburban East Keilor lies a small Mediterranean paradise. The only giveaways are the olive trees and a small wine barrel used as a post box on the nature strip. A few more steps take you on a side path around the back of the house and there you begin to have an idea of what Tony and Lina Siciliano have created in thirty-six years. The 7 acre property, which was in the beginning just a barren block of land with weeds and stones, has been transformed into a thriving small farm by Tony and Lina's passion, hard work and daring. What at the beginning was just a desire to grow some vegetables and plant fruit trees has become a lush and productive oasis in the middle of suburbia and a way of life for the Sicilianos.[1]

From Italy to Australia
Tony and Lina were born in Varapodio, a small town at the foot of the Aspromonte, the mountain chain in the Calabria region in the

south of Italy, famous for olive and citrus trees. Their family were farmers and life was hard, especially after the Second World War, and many people from Varapodio migrated to Australia, including Tony in 1963. He worked in various jobs, establishing himself in his trade as a painter, decorator and electrician. Like many young migrant men who left loved ones behind, he felt the separation from his fiancée, Lina, still in Varapodio. Tony went back to Italy in April 1965 and married the seventeen-year-old Lina in August. After their honeymoon, they sailed for Melbourne, Australia, in December 1965.

Tony was very successful in his trade, while Lina, despite missing her family, soon settled in the new land. They lived a comfortable suburban life raising their three children. However, Lina, who had grown up with a strong connection to the land thanks to her mother's teachings, yearned for a life more in tune with nature like the one she had left behind. She dreamt of land to keep chickens and to grow fruit trees and vegetables as she used to do in her home town. Finally, in 1981 when Tony retired, they found the right land in East Keilor. It was the beginning of Lina's dream, which also became Tony's and their children's. Today, after only three-and-a-half decades, many mature trees, a vineyard, an orchard and an extensive vegetable garden have been successfully established. They have created a productive and beautiful environment where seasonal food is enjoyed as soon as it is picked and traditional Calabrian traditions are observed.

Rose Creek Estate
Rose Creek Estate is laid out on three levels so that it can make the most of the land, which slopes down to Rose Creek, a small tributary of the Maribyrnong River. Walking down from the road, you find yourself on a terrace lined with orange, olive, pomegranate, walnut and nectarine trees, partially sheltered by a pergola covered by a Fox Grape vine *(Vitis Labrusca),* also called *uva fragola* (strawberry grape) in Italian. This vine is grown mostly for sentimental reasons and for the strong sweet aroma from the pretty white bunches of grapes hanging amongst the foliage. Tony and his son Angelo make a sparkling red wine from this grape called Fragolino. Every inch of the property has been planted and, as the terrace continues by the side of the house, more trees and plants join the ever-present olive trees and

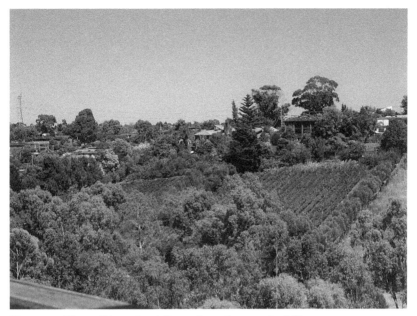

Figure 2.1. View of Rose Creek Estate from the opposite hill. Photo courtesy of Gabriella Gomersall-Hubbard.

Mediterranean herbs. Lina likes to experiment with exotic plants, so here are ice-cream beans, avocados, tamarillos, limes, babacos and even coffee trees; all doing fine next to elderberry, bay leaf, pomegranate, and citrus trees.

Citron and bergamot trees are grown not only for their fruit but also for their special connection with Tony and Lina's home town of Varapodio. They were the first citrus trees to appear in the Mediterranean Basin in the fourteenth century and have been grown successfully ever since in the Calabrian region, especially near Varapodio. In the eighteenth century, making bergamot snuff boxes became a traditional local craft, which continues even today. Neither fruit is edible, but they are still grown for their fragrant oil used in perfumery, aromatherapy or, as in the case of citron, confectionery. Another tree that Tony and Lina are emotionally attached to is the jujube, also called Chinese date or, in Calabrian dialect, *zinzuli* (*giuggiule* in Italian). The jujube is a graceful, ancient and nutritious tree not very well-known in Australia, but well-known in Asia for its medicinal properties and also common in Calabria. The little

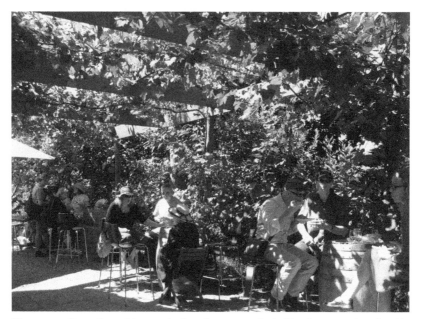

Figure 2.2. Open Day visitors enjoying the terrace shaded by fox grape (*uva fragola*). Photo courtesy of Gabriella Gomersall-Hubbard.

oval fruits are harvested in March and are rich in vitamins, minerals and antioxidants. Other interesting plants like pepino, prickly pear, comfrey, and angelica, as well as nut and fruit trees, including walnuts, plums, tamarillo, mulberry, quince, white sapote and even palm trees and bananas also grow along paths here and next to the olive trees.

The vineyards

Even from the terrace you can't really see the whole of the property now that trees have grown. Guarded by two cycad plants, a flight of wooden steps takes you down the hillside where two glorious green vineyards are revealed. Rows and rows of grapevines shine in the sun, completely protected by netting to defend them from the thieving birds. Initially, Tony planted the vineyard on the west side, then some years later when he was able to acquire more land, he planted the east vineyard. All together there are 3200 vines of different varieties: Merlot, Cabernet-Sauvignon, Shiraz, Semillon, Chardonnay, Pinot Noir, Cabernet Franc and the Italian variety Zibibbo. In the beginning, Tony was not sure whether the land would be suitable for

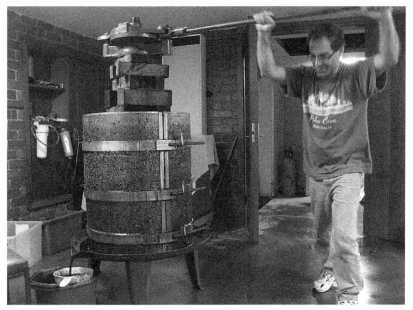

Figure 2.3. Angelo Siciliano making wine using a hand press. Photo courtesy of Gabriella Gomersall-Hubbard.

growing grapes, but the good fertile soil, the favourable position on the hillside, the water supply from Rose Creek and Tony's constant care have proved the right combination.

One crucial factor in this success story is the decision to adopt the Scott Henry trellis system developed by the American rocket scientist and viticulturist Scott Henry. The sturdy frames provide better sun exposure, higher yield and fewer diseases. Four canes are planted closely together: two are trained to an upper wire and two to the lower wire, leaving a space in the middle for wind and air. The system doubles the number of vines planted per metre and, although it is labour intensive, it is ideal for a small winery where grapes are handpicked. April is generally grape harvest time, an extremely busy time for the family and friends who come to help. It is important to pick the grapes when they have the right sugar content to produce wines with the right alcohol content. Every day, Tony and his son Angelo measure the sugar level in the grapes until the right amount is reached, hoping that this will coincide with favourable weather conditions for the harvest. Experience, intuition and the weather forecast play an important part in deciding when to pick the grapes in order to produce the best possible wine. While Tony grows and looks after the vines, Angelo is the winemaker. In the beginning, they used to sell their white and red grapes to other winemakers, but in 1994 Angelo decided to study winemaking at the Box Hill TAFE and at the Oakridge Estate. Since then, Tony's passion and knowledge, complemented by Angelo's expertise and professional approach, have produced fantastic results. Rose Creek Estate wines have been winning gold, silver and bronze medals and awards ever since.[2]

Opposite the western vineyard, the orchard provides an abundance of fruit each season: peaches and nectarines, lemons and oranges, walnuts and chestnuts, persimmons, cherries and, amazingly, tasty figs. Lina and Tony love their seventeen fig trees and protect them from the birds with high nets.

Keeping chickens

No Mediterranean garden would be complete without chickens. Lina has twenty to thirty chickens of different breeds, such as Leghorn, Gray Silkie, Silver and Gray Faverolles, Polish Bearded Buff, Isa Browns and many cross-breeds. There is also a rooster, two Guinea Fowls and two peacocks. They all live happily in a long and shady chicken run. Keeping chickens was always a long-held dream of Lina's and now they are not just kept for their eggs, but are regarded as pets. They lay an average of twelve eggs a day during the producing season and six to eight the rest of the year. 'They love pasta', says Lina, who also feeds them kitchen scraps and soy meal mixed with sunflower seeds, corn, maze, wheat and fresh greens from the vegetable garden.

The olive grove

It is autumn, the grapes have been picked, the wine just made, the weather is getting cooler and it is time to pick the olives. Lina and Tony grew up amongst the olive groves of Varapodio, a town that prides itself on its ancient and beautiful olive trees. They are very important to Lina and Tony and their way of life. They could not enjoy their tomatoes or beans or any other produce without extra-virgin olive oil; they could not cook or eat without it. Four hundred trees were planted around the property as a windbreak soon after Tony cleared

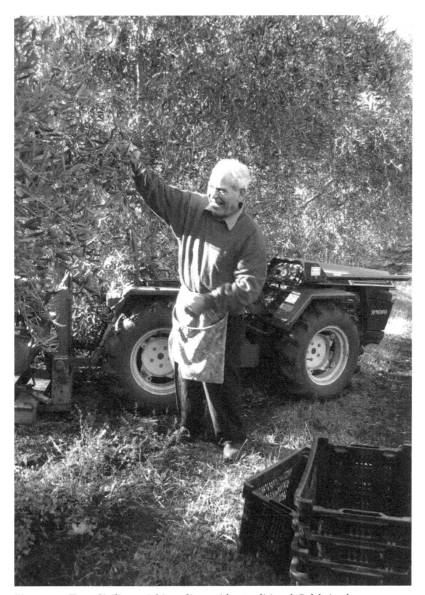

Figure 2.4. Tony Siciliano picking olives with a traditional Calabrian bag.
Photo courtesy of Gabriella Gomersall-Hubbard.

and fenced the land. There are several varieties: Corolea, Kalamata, Verdale, Correggiola, Frantoio, Spanish Queen and Manzanillo. Most of the olives are picked by hand and some are picked using a handheld tool that picks the olives without damaging the tree. It is intense and laborious work lasting many weeks. The most delicate moment is the pressing of the olives. Tony's olive press is a small machine bought in Italy which he has slowly modified, making improvements that have allowed him to produce a high-quality extra-virgin olive oil. Tony produces three kinds of extra-virgin olive oil: first harvest, made from green olives; second harvest, from semi-mature olives; and third harvest, from the mature olives. Rose Creek Estate first-harvest extra-virgin olive oil has a beautiful, intense emerald colour. Thanks to its fresh, peppery, fruity aroma and taste, it has won many awards, gold, silver and bronze medals and Champion category in numerous specialised competitions in Australia. Tony is, justly, very proud of what he has achieved. Over the years, he has become an expert in this field and his reputation has spread amongst the growers. A considerable part of his time is spent sharing his knowledge with others through demonstrations and one-on-one advice.

The vegetable gardens

If Tony is the expert on olive trees and vineyards and Angelo is the winemaker, Lina is the expert on vegetables and fruit trees (as well as the best cook). She has two vegetable gardens: one opposite the eastern vineyard by the big cypress tree and one in a new area on the west side of the property. They are quite extensive and their productivity is impressive. The plants are neatly planted in rows and are watered by a drip irrigation system set up by Tony. The water is drawn from the creek at the bottom of the land thanks to a permit obtained from the local council. Water is also stored in a tank which holds 60,000 litres as a reserve.

Summer and autumn are Lina's favourite seasons and are also when the vegetables are at their best. The red leaves of the amaranth contrast with the grey-blue Tuscan kale (*cavolo nero* in Italian), and the tomatoes, corn, eggplants, capsicum, red chillies, beans, cucumbers, zucchini and fennel thrive happily in neat rows. Edible flowers like nasturtiums, calendulas, zinnias, marigolds and dahlias grow amongst the vegetables and a great variety of herbs grows everywhere: basil, sage, rosemary, borage, Italian parsley, lemon balm, oregano, marjoram, thyme and the strong-scented rue – all of them find their way in corners and small spaces all over the property. Apple, walnut, peach, cherry and apricot trees also grow in this area.

Some of these vegetables are also grown in the western vegetable plot, as are a wide variety of beans. Tall and lush towers of beans grow row after row: green beans, Borlotti, Lima beans, butter beans and a particular variety from the home town of Varapodio: the Maddamola bean. A tobacco plant, grown for its beauty and as an insect repellent, grows next to another exotic plant originally from Chile and Peru. It is the *Physalis,* also known as husk-tomato or Cape gooseberry, which produces small Chinese-lantern-looking pods; their papery shells hide a surprisingly sweet little fruit. Growing splendidly is Tony's eggplant tree. It is really the Brazilian plant *Solanum Capsicoides* on which Tony has grafted three eggplant varieties: Violetta di Firenze, Bonita and a mini Lebanese. He has been very successful in growing and harvesting numerous healthy eggplants with this method. Rows of cantaloupe and watermelon grow next to tall Jerusalem artichokes, grown not only for their edible root but also for their bright yellow flowers. The new vegetable garden has given Tony and Lina the ability to grow more vegetables to take to the farmers markets. At the same time, Lina has organised all her crops in a cycle so vegetable seedlings are planted every two or three weeks to ensure that there is always something to harvest. Seedlings of eggplants, capsicums, African horn cucumbers, beans, tomatoes and other vegetables grow in various parts of the garden. Broccoli and broccoli rabe (or *cime di rape* in Italian), Jerusalem artichokes, red mustard, celery, silverbeet, garlic and onions are favourite winter crops, while broad beans, peas, lettuce and shallots are grown in spring.

The vegetable garden feeds the family all year round and is bountiful even in winter. It is here that Lina is happy tending the plants; it is here that Lina comes every day with her basket and her favourite knife to pick whatever is growing for the evening meal (see figure 2.5, colour insert). 'From the garden to the table' has real meaning in Rose Creek Estate. 'There is nothing as rewarding as growing, picking and eating your own food', says Lina, who cooks delicious food using the freshly picked vegetables and herbs. Her simple recipes handed down from her family are not only healthy but are also part of her Calabrian heritage.

Preserving

With so much seasonal produce, it is of the utmost importance to preserve the surplus. Lina carries on her Calabrian family tradition of bottling, drying and making sauces, sausages and salami. Not only does she regularly preserve the Kalamata olives in brine, but she also preserves fruit and vegetables. Borlotti and Maddamola beans are dried and kept in jars to be used in soups or salads. Little cucumbers and green beans are preserved in what Italians call *giardiniera* (garden vegetable mix). Herbs are dried in paper bags kept in the dark. Figs and tomatoes are dried in the sun and preserved in jars while others are strung together in attractive bunches and hung to dry next to bunches of red chillies. Some little tomatoes are, instead, placed in the freezer to be used when needed. At the centre of all this activity is the making of tomato salsa: *passata*. Lina and Tony's tomatoes have a wonderful aroma and taste, and preserving them is a cultural tradition at the centre of agricultural life in Italy. Making *passata* is a task that involves family and friends. Each person has a specific task to do, and time passes quickly telling stories and chatting while kilos and kilos of ripe red tomatoes end up in bottles and jars ready to be used during wintertime. The Calabria region is famous for its salami, sausages and other cured-pork products. Tony and Lina remember the ritual killing of the pig in the chilly winter months in Varapodio and, although they now buy the meat from a trusted butcher, they continue the tradition of salami and sausage making. Their salami, *capocollo* and pancetta are then smoked and hung from the rafters of the wood-oven shed, if the temptation to taste them can be overcome by the family, at least for a while.

Marketing and promotion: Markets and open days

Rose Creek Estate not only feeds the family, but also provides an income through the sale of its produce. What started as a family's passion has become a way of life and a profitable business. Three Saturdays a month, bottles of white and red wine and bottles of extra-virgin olive oil are taken to one of the farmers markets in the city to be sold at the

Rose Creek Estate stall, easily recognisable by the bright red umbrellas.[3] For sale also are olives in brine and fruit and vegetables arranged in pretty baskets. Sale of the produce is also available to customers (by appointment) at the estate, in the tasting room on the ground floor of the house, which was once the family's billiard room. Open days and participation at specialised events are also an opportunity to sell produce and to promote Rose Creek Estate, creating an invaluable network of contacts with people and organisations. In the past, open days were regularly held at the property in conjunction with Open Gardens Australia, the Sunbury Wine Festival and the Melbourne Food and Wine Festival, and were an opportunity to share with hundreds of visitors the paradise that the Sicilianos have created. After a tour of the estate, keen gardeners, families, foodies, young people and expert growers enjoyed simple and tasty food on the terrace by the side of the house with easy access to the tasting room. Although in recent years Lina and Tony have not held open days, they have continued to inspire people by welcoming gardening and Rotary clubs and small groups from various organisations interested in growing food or making wine or olive oil, such as the Stephanie Alexander Kitchen Garden Foundation, William Angliss students, local schools and Diggers Club members. They have participated in many festivals including the Tomato Festival, national Sustainable Living Festival, Lavandula Festival, Federation Festival and Darebin Homemade Food and Wine Festival.[4] Rose Creek Estate has been featured in many television programmes, such as *Food Safari*, *Vassili's Garden*, *Better Homes and Gardens*, *Family Food Fight* and the *Garden Tap*. The Sicilianos have also been featured in numerous publications and radio programmes. Lina has given cooking and preserving demonstrations, which end with a tasting of the delicious food prepared with her plants, to the delight of the participants.[5]

Rose Creek Estate: A sustainable paradise

Tony and Lina work hard all year round with some help from their children Maria and Angelo and some faithful friends. Through the years, they have shared their knowledge and practical approach with many people and have inspired others to grow their own food, but they have also learnt from others and have been not afraid to try new ways – the proof is in Rose Creek Estate's lush and bountiful crops.

In the beginning, their main concern was growing healthy food for their family, but they have become an example of how to live well, reduce our carbon footprint and care for the environment. Rose Creek Estate is organically managed, all crops are eaten fresh or dried, pickled or bottled, everything is biodegradable and recycled, and even the olive pips are returned to the soil. Pest and weed control is practiced through crop rotation and attention to the soil. Green manure crops and compost are used as fertilisers, as are chicken and cow manure and 'worm juice' from a small worm farm that Lina keeps near the chicken coop. These are complemented by blood and bone and seaweed concentrate. Seeds are saved from the family's favourite varieties of tomatoes, beans, broad beans and peas.

Tony and Lina's passion is evident not only in the high quality of produce, but also in the interesting diversity of plants and the beautiful landscape of the estate; they are proud of what they have achieved, but most of all they are happy to live in the paradise they have created in a corner of the city – a green oasis that reminds them of their home in Calabria.

Rose Creek Estate: The future

Tony and Lina, now in their early seventies, are still full of energy and enthusiasm. Their life is regulated by nature and the seasons and continues to be full and productive. The word 'retirement' is not in their vocabulary. Like many farmers, they have been working beyond the traditional retirement age.[6] The Australian Bureau of Statistics (ABS) Agricultural Census 2015–16 found that the average farmer is fifty-six years old, which is nearly 50% older than the average Australian worker at thirty-nine years old and is also more than the fifty-three years for the average farmer in the ABS's 2011 census. This is thought by some to be due to a decline in younger generations taking over the family farm, thanks to financial considerations or a desire to follow a different career path.

Farm succession is relevant not only to the family concerned, but it has global implications for food supply, as populations cultivating arable land diminish. The issue of farm succession has been receiving more attention, especially with regard to supporting young people to take up farming.

Passing on the family farm to the next generation is a difficult, delicate and emotional challenge, which not only Tony, Lina and their children face, but all farmers face. Succession is not easy to deal with and horror stories abound, but there are also success stories where the parents have chosen to discuss openly with their children the adoption of a succession strategy well before the occurrence of a crisis.[7]

Many farmers are not aware of the options available, such as share farming, leasing or joint-venture equity agreements, which will allow them to continue to live on the farm if they desire and at the same time provide a mentoring role to new farmers. Many agricultural experts advocate new and innovative ways to assist older farmers to transition into retirement and be recompensed, while remaining in contact with the agriculture sector.[8] Some of these ways have already produced successful community-supported agriculture models in many countries – a system that connects the producer and consumer, shares the risk of farming and produce, promotes sustainable agricultural practices and teaches skills. Some other organisations have set up a community land trust, which develops and preserves community assets on behalf of the community.[9]

Going back to the future of Rose Creek Estate, the conversation in Tony and Lina's family is ongoing. They look to the future with optimism, hoping that they will be able to care for Rose Creek Estate as long as possible. They are confident that 'when the time comes' they will reach a satisfactory decision about the future of the estate. They hope that the property will continue to produce wholesome food and to be an inspiration for people to live off the land. Most of all they hope that the urban 'paradise' they have created will be retained for future generations.

Acknowledgement

I have known Tony and Lina Siciliano and their family for ten years. Their knowledge and passion in establishing Rose Creek Estate has not only been a source of constant admiration and inspiration, but has also prompted me to write *Growing Honest Food*, a book about their life on the land. Month by month, season after season I have followed them in their daily chores in the estate, sharing their work, recording their knowledge and taking an active part in activities, cooking demonstrations, open days and related events. Their way of life has highlighted the beauty of the natural world and it is not only a healthy way to provide for oneself but is also a rewarding way to reduce our national and individual ecological footprints.

Chapter 3

Bringing Together Landless Farmers and Unused Farmland: The Sunraysia Burundian Garden and Food Next Door Initiative

Olivia Dun, Deborah Bogenhuber, Lesley Head,
Joselyne Kadahari, Natascha Klocker, John Niyera and
Joel Sindayigaya

This chapter tells the story of the Sunraysia Burundian Garden, a one-acre farm plot in Mildura Rural City. Here, members of a grassroots local food movement, Sunraysia Mallee Ethnic Communities Council (SMECC), Sunraysia Produce (a local fruit and vegetable wholesaler and retailer) and university academics have collaborated with members of Mildura's Twitezimbere Burundian Community to grow culturally important crops. This project and its associated Food Next Door (FND) initiative, established in 2016, emphasise sustainable food production and strengthened social ties as key ingredients of a more resilient food system and community.

Mildura Rural City: Food insecurity in an Australian food bowl
Mildura Rural City lies at the heart of the Sunraysia region where the Murray and Darling Rivers meet (figure 3.1). This semi-arid region has a population of approximately 64,000 people.[1] Historically, the rivers provided resources that enabled local Indigenous groups to settle with relative permanency.[2] In the late-nineteenth century, drought stimulated interest in irrigation and Mildura was established as one of Australia's

first irrigation settlements.[3] Over subsequent decades, Mildura's landscape came to be dominated by large-scale horticultural production.

Highly dependent on irrigation water, the Sunraysia region currently produces almost all of Australia's dried vine fruits (98 per cent) and table grapes (75 per cent), as well as significant volumes of almonds, pistachios, olive oil and citrus.[4] Recent commercialisation and expansion of vegetable farms has seen the region's growers now producing 13 per cent of Australia's carrots, alongside zucchini, squash, pumpkins and asparagus.[5]

Notwithstanding these high levels of fruit and vegetable production, a 2013 study found that a large number of residents in the Mildura municipality were 'food insecure'. In particular, they faced difficulty accessing locally grown, affordable fruit and vegetables. The

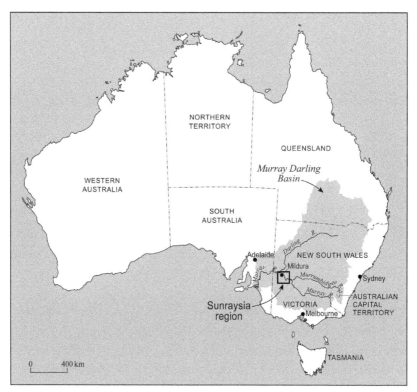

Figure 3.1. Location of Mildura within the Sunraysia region, which lies within the Murray Darling Basin and covers parts of north-western Victoria and south-western New South Wales. Map by Chandra Jayasuriya.

report attributed food insecurity to Mildura's relative disadvantage, as measured by social wellbeing, health, employment, economic and education indicators. It also signalled the significance of systemic barriers to the local availability of healthy food, including:
- poor market prices for local produce, encouraging farmers to export fresh produce rather than sell locally;
- difficulty accessing financially viable markets for produce, forcing smaller-scale farmers to leave the land;
- the lack of a central access point or coordinated activities to capture and re-distribute excess produce from local growers to local consumers;
- the high cost of fresh food for local consumers;
- the prevalence of takeaway food outlets in the Mildura food landscape: in 2013, there was only one dedicated greengrocer (Sunraysia Produce) in Mildura municipality, but seventy-one takeaway food outlets; and
- growth in export-oriented agribusinesses, especially around almond and table-grape production.[6]

Opportunities for farmland and farm work have long attracted migrants to the region. Consequently, it is one of Australia's most ethnically diverse rural areas: at least one-third of horticulturalists speak a language other than English at home.[7] Furthermore, in 2002, the Mildura local government area was declared a Refugee Welcome Zone[8] and refugees are increasingly settling in the area. A 2013 food security study found that 'many individuals and families from CALD [culturally and linguistically diverse] backgrounds have difficulty accessing culturally appropriate foods locally', with some travelling over 400 kilometres to Melbourne or Adelaide to access them.[9] It further identified that other than occasional farmers markets around the region, there were very few community events using food to bring people together and promote community ties.[10]

A local food movement
Against this backdrop of food insecurity, and with seed funding from the Victorian State Government, a local community food movement was started in Mildura in early 2016. Deb Bogenhuber, a leader of

Slow Food Mildura, received funding as a local food activator and initiated local food gatherings to open informal conversations with fellow community members. Deb was keen to understand their aspirations for the local food system and invited attendees to share their motivations for attending gatherings and explain what mattered to them.

Within a matter of months, the stories being told by those attending the food gatherings, together with results from a community survey, revealed a strong desire to see more small-scale farmers in the region, an increase in produce grown locally without the use of toxic chemicals and better access to locally grown food. Overall, a strong vision for the region emerged: a vision for the many under-utilised blocks in the irrigation district to be revitalised through small-scale regenerative farmers growing diverse abundant crops for the local community.

The local food movement grew to include Slow Food Mildura, community members with farming expertise and local small businesses. At the centre of the movement was a core group of around ten people who regularly attended local food gatherings and set about brainstorming, with optimism and energy, how the vision could be achieved. The diversity of this core group – born and bred locals and 'blow-ins', farmers and professionals, women and men, young and old(er) – generated innovative ideas. One of these was to identify underutilised land and 'match' it with people who wanted to grow food but did not have access to land.

Under-utilised farm blocks ready for rejuvenation

Since 2008–09, one quarter of irrigated cropland in the Sunraysia region had been left deliberately unirrigated as a consequence of the 1995–2009/10 drought, as well as due to other major social, economic and political factors.[11] The federal government had issued one-off grants encouraging 'small block' (<40 hectares) farmers to exit production (i.e. cease irrigation) for at least five years. Large areas of land were left 'dead, bare or barren'[12] (figures 3.2a, b). By the mid-2010s, the five-year irrigation ban on these blocks was ending, so efforts were underway to replant and rejuvenate approximately 1700 'dry blocks' in the Sunraysia region.[13] This particular confluence of events meant that there was land in need of (new) farmers.

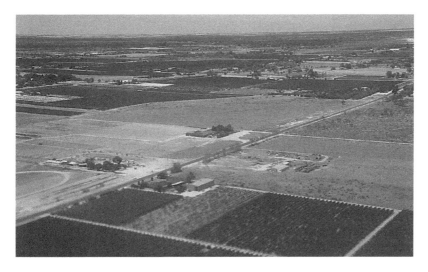

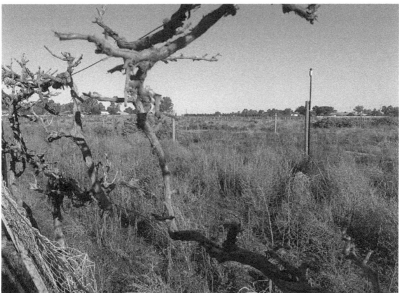

Figures 3.2a and 3.2b. Examples of under-utilised farm blocks in Mildura (photos taken in 2014 and 2017, respectively). Photos courtesy of Olivia Dun.

Landless farmers and former refugees in search of farmland

Parallel to the formation of the local food movement and the desire to rejuvenate dry blocks, a team of academics (Head, Klocker and Dun) was conducting research with migrant and refugee communities in the Sunraysia region under the 'Exploring culturally diverse perspectives on Australian environments and environmentalism' project.[14] Since 2014, the research team, helped along by SMECC, had been interviewing diverse community members to better understand how migrants' environmental understandings and capacities have shaped agricultural practices in the region. Among those interviewed were members of Mildura's Burundian community, comprising approximately nineteen families or 100 people in all.[15]

Eight members of the Burundian community were interviewed in October 2015. At that time, they had been living in Mildura for between one and five years. Many families had relocated to Mildura of their own accord after spending time living in larger Australian cities. They had a range of motivations for moving to Mildura, including the possibility of farming. Joel Sindayigaya, the president of Mildura's Twitezimbere Burundian Community Association, recalled his first impressions of Mildura: 'I looked around and saw…this town is a town of farmers… The happiest thought was to see the thriving farms. I said, "This place is good for me. There is something here".' This suite of interviews revealed that almost all adult members of Mildura's Burundian community had been farm owners in their country of origin and/or had farmed for several years while based in refugee camps in other African countries.

Despite being experienced farmers, none of the interviewees were farm owners in the Sunraysia region, primarily because they could not afford to rent or purchase farmland. Through the interview process, they expressed an overwhelmingly strong desire to farm in Australia. They wanted to grow food for subsistence/food security (and eventually for sale), to gain access to culturally important foods, to improve their physical and mental health, reduce isolation and inactivity, and to build connections and create a sense of belonging. They saw an opportunity to put their farming skills and experience to use in the Sunraysia landscape, but lacked access to land: they were landless farmers. During the research interviews, Joel asked the researchers, 'is there any way possible to bring a request forward about how people [in our Burundian community] might be able to receive help to have something to do, like farming...?'

Food Next Door is launched

Armed with this request from the Burundian community, and aware that there were many unused farm blocks dotted around Mildura, the research team organised a workshop to bring together diverse stakeholders from the horticultural, social service, and educational sectors in the Sunraysia region. The 'Diverse people, diverse crops: Exploring agricultural possibilities in the Sunraysia' workshop, convened in partnership with SMECC and Mildura Development Corporation, was held on 12 May 2016 at SMECC premises. The main objectives were for the research team to outline their findings and to identify possibilities to develop and implement a small-scale pilot project to match newer refugee and migrant arrivals with unused (or under-utilised) farmland.

Joel spoke on behalf of the Burundian community. He asked for help to access around 4 acres of farmland. Fortuitously, Deb and other members of the local food movement were present at the workshop. They explained their recent efforts to identify parcels of unused farmland that could be used to grow local food for the local community. Despite having identified appropriate plots of land, they had been unable to find growers with both farming skills and time to spare. While the research team had identified landless farmers, the local food movement had identified farmerless land!

Immediately following the workshop, a meeting was convened between the research team, Deb and Sunraysia Produce (also a local food movement member), who confirmed that they were happy to provide the Burundian community with free access to one acre of farmland adjacent to their business. This moment kick-started the Sunraysia Burundian Garden, the inaugural pilot demonstration of the Food Next Door model, an initiative (then unnamed) that matches landless farmers with unused land.

The Sunraysia Burundian garden sprouts and grows

By September 2016, only four months after the workshop, the Burundian community was sowing maize seeds. Key to this success was the high priority placed on regular, ongoing communication and clarification of expectations between the various parties.

Shortly after the workshop, an initial site visit was arranged for Burundian community members to see the land and meet the owners of Sunraysia Produce. This meeting was facilitated by Deb and the research team. Discussions focused on how the site could be used, what could be grown and any particular preferences or non-negotiable issues for all parties involved. A crucial point of compatibility, also key to the success of the pilot, was that the Burundian community preferred to grow their food without use of synthetic chemicals. This was a top priority for Sunraysia Produce, who otherwise placed no restrictions on what food could be grown or methods used.

Subsequently, Deb facilitated the development of a Memorandum of Understanding (MoU) between the Burundian community and Sunraysia Produce.[16] Through this process, a relationship developed between these two unlikely partners, based on mutual respect and trust. The MoU set out the purpose of the garden, as well as the expectations, roles and responsibilities of each party, insurance policies, timelines and review procedures.

Financial support was extremely limited; however, the Sunraysia Burundian Garden benefited from many other forms of support. Between signing the MoU and sowing the first maize seeds, several local food movement members volunteered their time and equipment, working together and forming relationships with the Burundian community as they prepared the land. The land was cleared of old wire, posts and fencing, slashed and rotary hoed with the help of Dean, a sixth-generation wheat farmer, and his tractor. The land was fenced by a local Indigenous environment team. A load of worm castings was donated by Australian Vermiculture (a local business), while a load of manure and 'African-like' garden hoes were purchased with the Burundian community's own funds. Once the land was prepared, an official opening was held, with speeches by Deb and members of the Burundian community (see figure 3.3, colour insert). This ceremony was important. It acknowledged the generous donations of time,

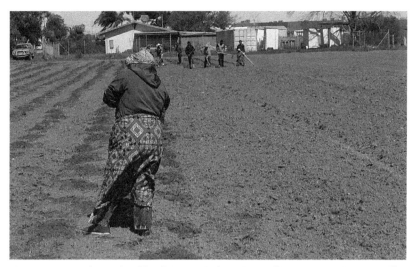

Figure 3.4. Members of Mildura's Twitezimbere Burundian Community manually sowing maize seeds at the Sunraysia Burundian Garden in September 2016. Photo courtesy of Olivia Dun.

equipment, resources and land received. By bringing people together it showed the Burundian community how much support they had from within the broader community. Equally, it enabled members of the broader community to become engaged in the first project of this kind in the Sunraysia region.

The Burundian community then took full leadership of the project, sowing their maize and bean seeds and integrating manure and worm castings according to their own deft and speedy manual methods. While irrigation equipment and a diesel pump were subsequently donated and installed with the help of the local food movement team, the Burundian community took responsibility for maintaining a watering and weeding regime as they tended to their crops. As the maize grew, some locals were sceptical as to whether the infamous Johnson grass could be kept at bay without weedicides. However, through their preference and capacity to farm as a group, the Burundian farmers kept the weeds under control manually. By January 2017, a maize crop stood tall in Mildura, impressing many locals who were delighted to see a previously dry block become green again. In February 2017, a harvest barbecue attracted members of the local community wanting to taste this new 'local' crop (see figure 3.6, colour insert).

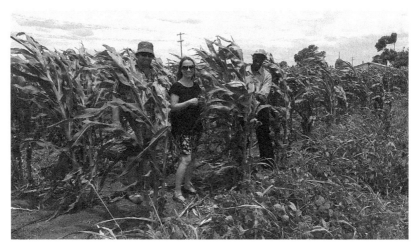

Figure 3.5. Joel shows Dean (Food Next Door member) and Natascha (research team member) the Burundian community's maize crop in January 2017.
Photo courtesy of Olivia Dun.

Contributions towards community resilience and sustainability of food systems: some reflections

The pilot demonstration, established without an instruction manual and with virtually no financial support, ran for approximately twelve months. It was successful owing to the hard work, joy and commitment to farming shown by the Burundian community; in-kind contributions; a local community's willingness to make a shared vision happen; and crucial support from the broader local food movement in Australia, particularly in Victoria, via a sharing of values and knowledge. This pilot offered an entirely new opportunity for locals to act on issues that concerned them. Through extensive media coverage[17] and the garden's highly visible city location, it demonstrated to the broader Mildura community what is possible in a place where locals are often heard saying that 'nothing much happens'.

Despite the uniqueness of the garden in Mildura, there were many commonalities with metropolitan-based urban agriculture initiatives: resources were scarce, activities were driven by the grassroots and were underpinned by a shared desire to create an alternative food system.[18] As such, the Sunraysia Burundian Garden contributes to the ever-increasing number of, often community-led, urban agriculture initiatives in Australia. Somewhat distinctively, however, the Sunraysia

Burundian Garden is a grassroots urban agriculture initiative in a rural setting. The stark evidence of supermarket chains' impacts (in terms of inhibiting access to locally grown fresh produce) is perhaps even more visible in Mildura than in larger cities. Mildura locals can literally see fresh produce being grown all around them, or are themselves involved in growing it or labouring on the land, but still cannot readily access locally grown fruit and vegetables. This unique context perhaps brought an unlikely combination of community members together around an urban garden initiative. The involvement of farmers in the Sunraysia Burundian Garden (including established local farmers and experienced farmers from the Burundian community) triggered new ideas among the local food movement for how broader-scale changes to the food system might be achieved and about the importance of migrants and refugees in this vision. What commenced as a project connecting diverse people through food and providing clear social and wellbeing benefits for the Burundian community, may yet have broader economic and political implications.

The pilot project has prompted the expansion of Mildura's local food movement into a much larger initiative that aspires to continue connecting landless farmers with under-utilised farmland. During the establishment of the Sunraysia Burundian Garden, the core group of local food movement members formed a not-for-profit cooperative, Food Next Door (FND).[19] FND is an organisation that seeks to build community through food and to advance the vision for a revitalised local food system Australia-wide. Two positions on the FND board are held by members of the Burundian community. The next stage involves establishing a community demonstration farm – where members of the Burundian community and FND can mentor other new migrants to the region and support them to grow diverse crops on donated farmland. This dream has already engaged broader institutions in the Sunraysia region and beyond, including local and state government agencies and authorities, local businesses, educational institutions and not-for-profit groups. If successful, it will provide yet a further example of an alternative farming model for Australia.

For Burundian community members, the pilot project provided a chance to demonstrate their farming knowledge and skills, culminating in a successful maize harvest. It also enabled them to grow a culturally important crop and to share this food with others, while creating a sense of well-being, belonging and a positive outlook. It provided insights into Australia's food-growing sector and potential business opportunities (e.g. via the milling of maize into flour) and connected the Burundian newcomers with long-term residents of Mildura in ways that evolved into lasting friendships.

Now that the pilot phase has ended, the Burundian community continues to grow food on the pilot site and plans to commence trialling peanuts and African beans on another 4-acre plot in Mildura donated by a private land owner. They are also keen to farm on an even larger plot at the proposed FND community demonstration farm. The future of all these activities is uncertain, contingent on funding, resources and availability of all those involved. What is not missing, however, is a sense of determination and enthusiasm amongst the Burundian community to continue to farm wherever opportunity allows. While the pilot and follow-on activities are still a fragile experiment with an uncertain future, they have served to highlight the increasing presence and role of migrants and cultural diversity in Australian rural towns, and the ways in which farming can effectively create a sense of belonging for such migrants.

Addendum

The authors are very pleased to note that Food Next Door's community demonstration farm was put forward as a priority for the Mallee region under the Victorian Government's Regional Partnerships model, which is a consultative approach for engaging closely with Victoria's regions. This model recognises that local communities are in the best position to understand the challenges and opportunities faced by their regions. Just as this chapter went to press, we were notified that the Victorian Government will provide over half a million dollars in funding to support Food Next Door's activities. The next step in this story will be the development of a project plan that details the establishment phase of the Food Next Door community demonstration farm over the next three years. This will enable the Food Next Door team to support more migrants, former refugees and otherwise marginalised groups to access farmland and to practice regenerative farming.

Affiliations and acknowledgements

This chapter represents a collaboration between authors from a range of institutions and backgrounds: Olivia Dun is affiliated with the School of Geography, University of Melbourne, and the School of Geography and Sustainable Communities, University of Wollongong; Deborah Bogenhuber is with Slow Food Mildura and Food Next Door; Lesley Head is affiliated with the School of Geography, University of Melbourne; Joselyne Kadahari, John Niyera and Joel Sindayigaya are members of the Mildura Twitezimbere Burundian community; and Natascha Klocker is affiliated with the School of Geography and Sustainable Communities, University of Wollongong.

Numerous people and organisations need to be thanked for contributing their strengths and experience to make the Sunraysia Burundian Garden a success: Mildura's Twitezimbere Burundian community for their commitment, enthusiasm and leadership. Dianne Boston and Tony Trinick of Sunraysia Produce for their complete generosity of spirit and gutsiness in venturing into the unknown by providing farmland access to complete strangers. Local food movement members (particularly Reece Cameron, Ben Dunn, Sevilla Furness-Holland, Rachel Kendrigan, Dean Lampard, Tony Lyons, Tess Spaven and Peter Webb) for their multiple donations of volunteer hours, equipment, expertise and enthusiasm. Jennifer Douglas (Jenny) and Emma Brown for their wonderful ABC news and Landline reporting and Jenny's continued unfailing support for the Burundian community's farming endeavours. Brendon and Del Price and the team at Australian Vermiculture for their donation of worm castings. Peter Webb for his mentoring and training expertise in ecological farming practices. Fiona Bawden and Richard Mintern for hosting the Burundian community on-farm compost training workshop, including donations of diverse manure types. Rachel Kendrigan and Tess Spaven for working from the heart in their facilitation, documentation and coordination of garden events and milestones. Barkindji Maraura Elders Environment Team (BMEET) for their time and labour constructing a fence around the garden. A generous anonymous donor who contributed to covering water and irrigation costs. Dean Wickham of SMECC for a wonderful introduction to the Mildura Burundian community and steadfast support in highlighting the strength and abilities of Mildura's newly arrived and established migrant and refugee groups. Paul Mbenna for research assistance, translation and interpretation that went well beyond paid hours. Slow Food Mildura and Andrea Sloane for having the foresight to support 'local food activation' activities. Jenny Garonne (formerly of Mildura Development Corporation) for her strategic support. Pippa French and the team at 3000acres as well as Serenity Hill, Kirsten Larsen and the team at the Open Food Network for their technical and moral support. Mildura Rural City Council, UpStart Co-working space and Cristal Mining for their cash and in-kind contributions. Tony Alessi and Steve Timmis for their strategic support in relation to the evolving Food Next Door community demonstration farm. Finally, we thank Andrea Gaynor for her helpful editorial comments on earlier versions of this chapter. All of the research conducted in association with the Sunraysia Burundian Garden has been funded by the Australian Research Council Discovery Project 'Exploring culturally diverse perspectives on Australian environments and environmentalism' (DP140101165) and by internal research funds from the University of Melbourne, including the 'Diverse farmers, diverse crops' community engagement grant (MEGS20170034).

Chapter 4

Cultivating Community

Peta Christensen

Established in 1998, Cultivating Community is a Melbourne-based NGO working in urban agriculture and community food initiatives.[1] We work with people from many different cultural backgrounds mainly in low-income communities, which makes for a wonderful and fascinating exploration of relationships to food and the food system. Cultivating Community supports community gardens on public housing estates, delivers community composting and food waste reduction initiatives and runs school food-garden programs, a community food centre and activities on all things community food and food systems.

People, plants and culture

Most people recognise the public housing towers dotted around Melbourne's inner-city neighbourhoods; however, what most people don't know is that below many of those towers are thriving community gardens where people from over thirty language groups are growing their own food. These gardens are some of the most productive growing spaces you'll find, especially in the city, with gardeners from countries including Vietnam, China, Turkey, Sudan, Afghanistan,

El Salvador, Greece, Egypt and East Timor, making the most of every inch of their 2 metre by 2 metre plots.

Community garden plots provide so much more than a place to grow vegies; for many, these gardens are a sanctuary where they can relax and unwind, talk with friends or just be 'on their land'. Much of the food grown is highly culturally specific, often not readily available in the supermarkets or greengrocers. So being able to grow it yourself is essential to maintain the connection to culture and identity. Over the years, countless gardeners have told me their garden has saved their marriage or even their life — that having a little patch of land has provided the space to take a break from the difficulties of being newly arrived or unwell or not being able to speak English or being on a low income.

I first started volunteering with Cultivating Community in 2000 after hearing then Chairperson Greg Milne at the Woodford Folk Festival talk about the need to grow more food in cities. He spoke about Basil Natoli, who was raising the profile of the public housing community gardens with the aim of securing state government support. Basil's aim was to ensure these often-informal gardens could be resourced to provide a vital lifeline for the many people he had encountered in the gardens.

When I came to Melbourne I looked Basil up and started volunteering with him. His enthusiasm and commitment were infectious and I fell in love with these incredible spaces where some serious magic seemed to be happening. When I asked Basil how he began his journey with the public housing community gardens, Basil told me about a community garden meeting in Collingwood that was conducted entirely in Vietnamese.

At that time Basil, a horticulturalist and teacher, didn't even know what a community garden was. At one point in the meeting everyone turned to look at Basil and started cheering. Basil asked his colleague what was going on and he said they were all very happy because he was going to help them get a garden going. After seeing how joyful the prospect of a garden made everyone, how could he not do all he could to help make that happen? And so it began, with Basil learning Vietnamese at night school so he could talk to people about what they wanted and the process of building the garden.

Basil introduced the then Victorian Minister of Housing, Anne Henderson, to what was happening in these early community gardens. The minister was instantly impressed with what she saw and the people she met in the gardens. In Basil's words, 'the Minister's eyes were opened up to the extraordinary benefits the gardens were making to the lives of public housing residents'.

In the late 1990s, Cultivating Community (then known as Coll-LINK) was no longer able to attract funding to continue its work and went into a brief period of organisational hibernation.

Discussions with Anne Henderson led to Basil being invited to develop a long-term plan for public housing community gardens and, in 2000, Basil was employed as the first community gardens program manager of what we know today as the Department of Health and Human Services' Office of Housing. After almost a decade of lobbying the Victorian State Government about the importance of food growing and the recreational and therapeutic benefits of gardening for people living in high-rise public housing estates, Basil suddenly found himself in the key role overseeing the implementation of all the things he had been working for!

Soon after, Cultivating Community advertised for its first paid position working with kids, gardening on three different housing estates across Melbourne. I applied and was lucky enough to get the job. From here I went on to work in community gardens associated with public housing. In those days, it was all new – there were no how-to manuals, few existing projects and Basil and I were making it up as we went along.

In 2002, based on Basil's work, the Department of Human Services was seeking interest from groups to run an ongoing service supporting public housing gardens on sites such as Fitzroy, Richmond, Collingwood, Carlton, North Melbourne, Prahran and South Melbourne. The new Cultivating Community committee had extensive discussions about the implications of submitting for the tender, but it decided to take a big step and grasp the opportunity. It won the tender and on 20 June 2002 Cultivating Community signed the public housing community gardens contract. This contract and our public housing community gardens work remain in place today as a core part of what we do.

It wasn't long after spending time with Basil and the community gardeners that I began to see how emotionally and even spiritually connected to their gardens people were and how these small patches of land meant so much to people for so many reasons. Even now, nearly twenty years later, it's that connection that most inspires me about the work that we do.

Sometime in the early 2000s I was working in a small community garden in Collingwood when some of the gardeners became extremely concerned about a dispute that was rapidly escalating between two key garden members because one of the gardeners had pruned a peach tree that was in his neighbour's garden. The ill-placed tree had grown vigorously over the years from a stray seed to a substantial tree and was now overshadowing his plot. When the owner discovered the pruned tree, he became extremely distressed and enraged.

I'd never encountered a situation like this so I called Basil and we decided we had better do something immediately, otherwise who knew what would happen if we left things to unfold over the weekend. A hasty mediation session was called involving Vietnamese and Turkish interpreters and, after some loud and heated exchanges, both men were almost in tears, one lamenting the damage done to the beautiful tree he described as being like one of his children and the other saying he had prayed to take back his actions because he was feeling so much remorse for hurting his friend. The men, through their respective interpreters, both acknowledged their deep respect for each other and were able to accept the mistake and move on.

I was incredibly moved by the deep connection these men had to each other and this patch of dirt through their shared love of gardening and, although they didn't speak the same language, they both profoundly understood the practice of turning up every day, every season, to lovingly tend their food gardens.

Around this time, Cultivating Community also partnered with Stephanie Alexander to establish a school food garden and cooking program at Collingwood College. Stephanie approached Basil with the idea, inspired by her friend Alice Waters in California who had started the Edible Schoolyard concept in 1995 to teach kids how to grow and cook their own food. School food gardens are still a big part of our work, teaching children about growing food, getting

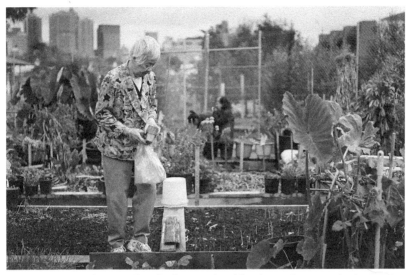

Figure 4.2. New shoots and fresh plantings herald a change in season in the Highett St Community Garden, Richmond. Photo courtesy of Rachelle Davey.

their hands dirty and connecting with the natural world. This kind of education is invaluable, and hopefully we're teaching the kinds of skills that will benefit these kids throughout their lives, whether it be growing a food garden, composting or just understanding a bit more about where our food comes from. We also see that these gardens can be an integral part of a community food system, potentially providing multiple ways for people across the community to be involved. As they are natural community hubs, usually centrally located and often with great facilities that are only used during school hours, there is still much to be explored in order to maximise this potential.

A few years later we started thinking more about the role community gardens played in terms of food insecurity, about how growing your own food could make a big difference to being able to access fresh, healthy and affordable food when you are on a low income. We also knew there were plenty of people living on the estates who didn't have a plot in the gardens and who had difficulty getting to the shops or found fresh food in the supermarket to be too expensive. In 2004, we partnered with the Brotherhood of St Laurence to pilot a fresh food community market on the Fitzroy Estate. The idea was to set up a volunteer-run market close to where people lived, selling seasonal produce with as little mark up as possible. Most of the produce was sourced from the wholesale fruit and veg market, however, some was grown in our community gardens or donated from local gardeners. Volunteers gained skills and confidence in working in the enterprise (as well as getting a box of produce each week) and local people shopped with their neighbours getting great-value fresh produce as well as getting to know each other a little bit more. Anne, one of our key volunteers at the time, talked about how working at the market meant that she now knew everyone and would chat to people in the lift she never would have spoken to before. We started a second market on the Collingwood Estate and delivered that program for a number of years before the pressures of running an extremely lean community-food enterprise became too tough. We're so pleased that another community food organisation, the Community Grocer, has refined and tweaked this market model, successfully running no less than six markets across Melbourne!

We were also thinking more and more about peak oil and climate change and the role of urban agriculture in relation to food systems thinking, as well as the need to build resilient communities in preparation for future resource stresses. We applied to the City of Yarra, a local inner-city municipality in Melbourne, for funding to initiate a number of community food projects, including a local community food group who worked on an early version of a food policy and also started a local food swap. The food swap idea was based on the CERES City Farm's Neighbourhood Orchard, a formalising of the age-old concept of swapping and sharing your excess produce with your neighbours. The Fitzroy Urban Harvest group decided to meet on the first Saturday of the month at a local park: the rules were simple, you brought what you could and took what you needed. People certainly brought loads of stuff but it did take a little while for people to feel okay about taking stuff; the concept of free food was uncomfortable for many. The quantity and variety of produce landing on the swap table was amazing, sometimes seeing up to 90 kilograms move through the swap in just two hours and featuring local delicacies like Japanese raisins, Fitzroy macadamias and quail eggs.

The success of the Fitzroy Urban Harvest Food Swap has been largely due to the irrepressible energy and passion of the late, great

Glenda Lindsay, a tireless local community food advocate who will long be remembered for her innovative ideas, bulldog-like tenacity, constant lobbying, colour and flair. It was through many a conversation at the food swap that ideas like Compost Mates was born as a way to reduce food waste going to landfill from local cafes and create compost for local gardens. What started with a team of gardeners collecting scraps from three local cafes soon expanded through a number of iterations to become Food Know How, a Melbourne-wide program working across five local council areas with a focus on food waste avoidance – an excellent example of the capacity of community food projects to address complex community issues.

A few years ago, we were approached to run a program in a basic but lovely, light-filled kitchen attached to our Fitzroy community garden. We started with a community lunch group, which soon evolved into an after-school cooking program so the participants could involve their kids in learning to cook. The obvious, yet wonderful connection between garden and kitchen opened up a whole world of community food possibilities and we looked to the Canadian Community Food Centres model for inspiration to further increase ways to bring people together around growing, cooking, sharing and advocating for nutritious and sustainable food. Our Fitzroy Community Food Centre complements our community garden perfectly as it provides a place for people from both our community garden and the broader community to come together around food, whether it be a community lunch, cultural cooking group, bread baking or food-waste avoidance workshop, after-school cooking or using the kitchen for small food-enterprise development. This simple, yet dynamic space has shown us the many community food possibilities that a garden and kitchen can nurture, and we are now extending these community food activities to the other estates where we are working with support from the Lord Mayor's Charitable Foundation, which has been instrumental in supporting Cultivating Community in exploring new projects and ideas.

A national perspective

In 2002, after countless phone calls and enquiries from people wanting to know about how they could get involved with or start a community garden in their neighbourhood, Cultivating Community decided to put together what we called the Green Map. We aimed to pull together a resource showing all of the community gardens and school-garden projects across Melbourne. We managed to map around sixty projects, knowing there were quite a few more gardens out there that we didn't know about. It was around this time that we also started connecting with other people across the country who were involved with community gardens and food projects, including those who were part of what was to become the Australian City Farms and Community Gardens Network (ACFCGN), a national voluntary community group whose aim is to connect people interested in community food-growing initiatives across the country.

According to Russ Grayson, ACFCGN started in the summer of 1994 when he and Fiona Campbell organised a meeting to gain an idea of the extent of community gardening in Sydney. They knew about a number of projects, including Glovers Community Garden (Sydney's first community garden, established in 1985 and still going today), Angel Street Permaculture Garden, in inner-city Newtown, and Randwick Community Organic Garden, but they were curious about what else was out there.

Russ and Fiona thought perhaps a dozen or so would come to the meeting, but when around thirty-five to forty people turned up they realised something significant was happening – they just weren't sure what it was!

Darren Phillips, then a student at ANU, came along to the meeting. He was researching community gardens and what he described as community 'enterprise centres'. After the meeting, he suggested they needed a network to share information and advice, so the Australian City Farms, Community Gardens and Enterprise Centres Network was formed. Later the Enterprise Centres element was dropped and representatives from around the country were recruited to provide a contact point and information resource for the growing number of community garden projects across Australia.

Representing and connection this growing number of community gardens was and remains the group's main purpose. Early on, the network aimed to have community gardening recognised as a valid urban land use, and later the mission grew to include consulting and advocacy, supporting groups by providing information to help set up community gardens, develop decision-making, conflict resolution and communications strategies and also address the social design of community gardens.

By the early 2000s, the network had achieved its goal of having community gardening recognised as a valid urban land use, which was evident by the growing number of gardens in Australian cities. Around 2007, Russ Grayson wrote what we think was the first community gardening policy directions document for local government to enable the development of community gardening. Many municipalities have created similar strategies and policies across the country since then and many more continue to follow suit recognising the multi-dimensional value of growing food in the city.

It's heartening and exciting to reflect on the growth of community food growing projects across the country over the past twenty years – in a way, it's a natural extension of our fundamentally human desire to grow things, but taking it out of the backyard and into our city streets and public spaces creates a whole new level of food production and consciousness that just might be one of the critical things that helps us to remember our place in the cycle of all things.

PART 2

Permaculture, Sustainability and Resilient Urban Food Systems

Chapter 5

Unearthing the Potential of Home Food Production

Kat Lavers and Hannah Moloney

At a time when our cities are bursting at the seams with growing populations, it's become far more common to live in apartment buildings and townhouses. However, despite increasing urban density, much of the land in the suburbs remains devoted to gardens and, with them, one of Australia's favourite pastimes – gardening. What, then, is the role of the humble vegie patch today, and does it have a place in future food systems?

The current mainstream urban food system is centred around a supermarket duopoly in which food often travels tens of thousands of kilometres to reach us.[1] It's dependent on fossil fuels for production, packaging and transport, and highly vulnerable in the event of supply disruption. As experiences like the Brisbane floods in 2011 have demonstrated, breaks in the supply chain can mean empty supermarkets within a week. This system also lacks transparency and consumers have little, if any, knowledge of, let alone a relationship with, the people, the animals and the land that produces their food. But we know another system is possible. In this chapter, we explore what a more sustainable food system might look like, with a focus on the role of home food production.

Land

Let's start our journey with a large urban property, Good Life Permaculture. Located under 3 kilometres from Hobart city, this property is on just over 3000 m² on a steep, sunny hillside. Hannah, with partner Anton and daughter Frida (figure 5.1) used the permaculture design framework to design resilience and abundance into their landscape and lives. They grow all their perishable vegetables, have chickens for eggs, goats for milk, bees for honey and a range of fruit and nut trees at varying ages. They walk and graze their goats through the local weedy bush to provide diverse fodder and exercise. They cycle their nutrients onsite with composting toilets and food-waste composting and, while they're connected to mains water and electricity, they still harvest the sun with solar panels and rain with tanks. They renovated the house so more people could live onsite – maximising the house's potential and supplying affordable housing. While most people would move to a rural community to have a small farm, Hannah and her family are doing it on a smaller scale in the city for two key reasons. Firstly, in the city they're closer to a lot of their community, something that's important to them, and secondly, it's easy to use bicycles, public transport and feet as transport, instead of relying on a petrol guzzling car all the time.

It's not necessary, though, to have a large property, or even very secure tenure, to make a more self-sustaining home. While living in a small North Hobart property for six months from mid- to late 2012, Hannah and Anton managed to establish a vegetable garden and chicken system, diverting greywater from their laundry into the garden. Within a short amount of time they were producing around 50 per cent of their fresh food intake. As they had many years of experience behind them, they were able to establish a productive and beautiful garden within two weeks and spend the rest of their time there eating from it. To make this happen they had to talk directly to the landlord and convince him that they were capable, that the property wouldn't turn into a mess and that they would either return the space to lawn once they moved out or find a new tenant who was an avid gardener

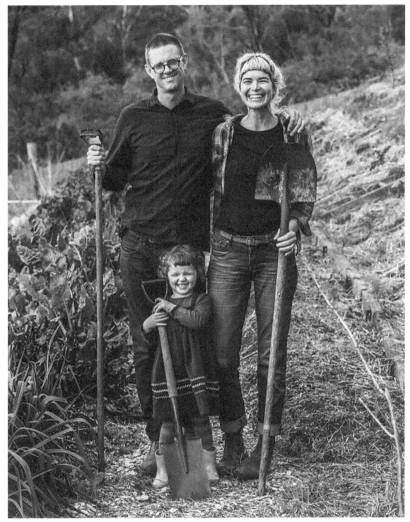

Figure 5.1. Anton Vikstrom, Hannah Moloney and Frida Vikstrom in the garden at Good Life Permaculture, Hobart. Photo courtesy of Natalie Mendham.

to take on the commitment of the garden. While at first the landlord was hesitant, Hannah and Anton simply explained that gardening was not optional for them – if he didn't let them garden, they wouldn't move in. Luckily, the landlord came around and soon he even started dropping off sacks of animal manure to add to the soil and herb cuttings to boost the garden. He was able to see that the changes were actually improving his property.

Kat's urban permaculture system, 'The Plummery', is on a 280 square metre block in the inner Melbourne suburb of Northcote. The garden has intensively managed, raised vegetable beds; perennial forest garden edges with fruit and nut trees as canopy and soft fruit understories; an outdoor seating area with a productive grape canopy; quail aviary; and greenhouse. All organic waste is recycled onsite through worm farms, a deep litter system (see below), composting toilet and chop'n'drop mulching. The old shed has been retrofitted into a light earth studio to accommodate guests, WWOOFers (Willing Workers on Organic Farms) and interns. With the exception of storage crops like pumpkins and potatoes, the garden produces almost all the household's veggies, herbs, fruit and eggs – more than 350 kilograms in 2016! (See figure 5.3, colour insert.) As these examples demonstrate, the suburbs have vast, untapped capacity to increase the resilience of our food system.

Evidently many Aussies desire a similar connection with their food and need little persuasion of the value of home food production. One study found that around 52 per cent of households are growing some food at home already, with another 13 per cent intending to start.[2] People grow food for all kinds of reasons: some because they enjoy the exercise, others because they want to garden with children. Despite this popularity, home food production suffers from a high turnover rate and relatively low yields.

What are some of the most significant barriers to home food production and how might they potentially be navigated? For many aspiring growers, the first challenge is securing access to sufficient and suitable land. One of the most persistent myths about urban food production is that it takes a large backyard (or even a farm) to produce a meaningful quantity of produce. It's surprising to learn that by some estimates as little as 108 square metres (9 metres by 12 metres) can produce a year's supply of fruit and vegetables for one adult in south-eastern Australia.[3] Unfortunately, ever-increasing house prices and high rents are making access to even small gardens a real challenge. We hope that longer-term rental contracts and changes to negative gearing will reduce speculative investments and provide more affordable housing. In the meantime, one solution is to have more people living on each property instead of only one person/couple/

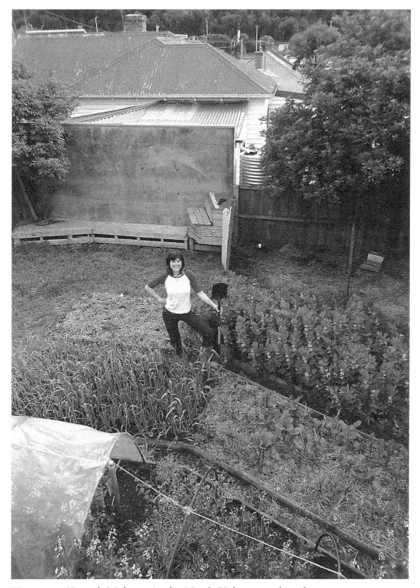

Figure 5.2. Hannah Moloney in the North Hobart rental garden, 2012.
Photo courtesy of Anton Vikstrom.

family. This could simply mean share housing or building tiny homes on your property to offer affordable, ethical housing to others.

Of course, as Hannah and Anton's example shows, you don't need to own land to grow food on it. We've both grown a significant contribution to our diet in rental properties and returned them to lawn at the end of our tenancy. Throughout urban spaces there are large areas of under-utilised fertile ground on public land, or areas that could be fertile with a bit of work. There's a huge opportunity for landholders (local government, business and private owners) to allow access to these areas for food production with medium- to long-term leases providing security of tenure to the growers. In Melbourne, not-for-profit 3000acres have helped many community groups negotiate tenure agreements with local government and other landowners. Here we are mainly concerned with food production at the household scale, but it's worth noting that the suburbs are full of public spaces, nature strips and disused blocks just waiting for a permaculture design and a bunch of enthusiastic community-minded folk to implement it.

When access to land is secured, the legacy of leaded petrol and paint often presents another challenge for home gardeners. Levels of lead (and other heavy metals) in soils around human settlements are in some cases elevated many times in excess of safe limits.[4] Fortunately, research consistently shows that in healthy soil, lead is not transferred into fruit in harmful quantities.[5] This means that fruit and nut trees, berries and vegetable 'fruits' like tomatoes and pumpkins are all good choices for sites with moderate contamination. Kat has managed lead at the Plummery with this and other strategies, including adding compost and mulch, maintaining soil pH at neutral or slightly alkaline, raising beds with clean imported soil for vegetables and washing produce to avoid accidental soil ingestion. The quail aviary is quarantined from the original soil to make sure heavy metals are not bio-accumulated in the birds and their eggs. Meanwhile, Hannah manages their lead-contaminated section of the garden by only growing fruit trees, natives and flowers in that area. While soil contamination is therefore a design consideration and can increase implementation costs for imported soil and raised beds, it's not an insurmountable barrier to food production.

Faced with the demands of a busy career and family commitments, it's not surprising that many people give up on the home vegie patch.

But how much time does it really take to manage a productive garden? At the Plummery, Kat is producing almost all the herbs, vegetables, fruit and eggs required for two adults and regular guests with about four hours' work a week on average. Gifting and swapping with friends and family has improved variety and supplied vegetables like pumpkins that need a larger growing area. Hannah spends around six to seven hours a week and supplies her family (two adults and a young child) with 90 per cent of their dairy, vegetables, honey and egg requirements as well as some fruit, and also regularly supplies their housemates and friends with produce.

In our experience, an hour or two a week would be more than enough time for most people's less ambitious production goals, but when viewed as one more activity to schedule into a crowded calendar, growing food at home can still be dismissed as too hard. Convenience is, however, a matter of perspective and time spent in the garden can replace time required for other tasks, like exercise or recreation. Hannah and Anton once took a season off growing vegetables while they tackled some building projects at home, but found shopping for food was a hassle and also felt their diet didn't have the same nutritional value. At the end of the season they declared that they'd never again go without a vegetable garden as it was simply too inconvenient.

Actual time management of serious home gardens tends to be considerably less than most people imagine, but the real-time barrier is the time it takes to start a garden and the time it takes to know how to start. Ultimately, we believe the most significant barrier to home food production may simply be a lack of skills, and this realisation has prompted us both to dedicate our lives to teaching.

Skills

In the context of busy lives and constraints like land availability, insecure tenure and soil contamination, it's important to design home food-production systems in a way that helps us make the most of available resources while working within these parameters. Our most valuable skill-set has been permaculture, a design framework based on universal ethics and principles that is used to create productive human settlements. Developed in Tasmania in the mid 1970s by Bill Mollison and David Holmgren, permaculture is now a global movement supporting people in moving away from dependence on fossil fuels towards a lifestyle that is resilient, connected and abundant. In a nutshell, permaculture creates 'consciously designed landscapes which mimic the patterns and relationships found in nature, while yielding an abundance of food, fibre and energy for provision of local needs.' [6] We can apply permaculture design at any scale, from a balcony garden on the tenth story of an apartment building to a quarter-acre block in the suburbs, and beyond.

So what does this look like in practice? In permaculture design we use functional integration and zoning to create energy-efficient gardens. For example, a 'deep litter' system is the result of functionally integrating chooks and compost. By placing a thick layer of carbon-rich materials, like wood shavings, on the base of the coop we are released from the chore of cleaning out stinky bird poo every week and we can simply harvest finished compost every few months. Zoning is another powerful tool for energy efficient design. Positioning herbs close to the house can mean the difference between a quick reach out the back door or walking the equivalent of several extra kilometres each year in regular trips down to the back garden (or more likely, giving up on fresh herbs with every meal). David Holmgren's *RetroSuburbia: A Downshifter's Guide to a Resilient Future*[7] documents the most promising permaculture strategies for south-eastern Australia following years of experimentation by ourselves and other practitioners.

We honed our skills by WWOOFing[8] alongside more experienced growers, Perma-blitzing and reading books, and we winnowed these lessons with plenty of good old trial and error, but today, there's an expanding list of resources for those wanting to rebuild this capacity. The internet is a phenomenal resource but, for growing food, local knowledge and observation of climate, soil and plants is essential. We happen to think that part of the joy of growing food is the gentle dance between the hope of planting, frustration of failure, attention of observation and learning, and the ultimate satisfaction of harvest. We gardeners cultivate soils, but we also cultivate our best selves! That said, online blogs and social media are an invaluable way to connect with local gardeners in the same bioregion and inevitably lead to swapping and sharing offline too.

In our experience, formal, locally based education projects can boost yields and also build community. Good Life Permaculture partnered with the Migrant Resource Centre and Sustainable Living Tasmania in 2014 to teach newly arrived refugees how to grow food in a cool temperate climate. We noticed that most refugees were being placed in the outer suburbs where some felt isolated and disconnected. Over a period of months, we worked with refugees from Afghanistan, Syria, Sudan, Uganda, Burma and Iran to turn their rental gardens into a haven of community and food productivity. While the project outcome was to build food gardens, the main aim was to build connections – which we did by playing soccer, listening to hip hop, eating and mucking around with all the kids.

The Home Composting Project was a collaboration between Good Life Permaculture and the City of Hobart Council in 2017. This multi-layered project was a creative education campaign that encouraged people to compost their food waste at home instead of sending it to landfill where it releases harmful methane gases into the atmosphere. There were three layers to this project. The first was focused on 'passive education' through installing large billboards throughout the city with stunning artwork and educational messages on composting (figure 5.4). The second layer involved 'active education', which took place through two free home-composting workshops in Hobart, where we worked with participants to collect data about how much food waste they composted at home. The third layer was advising the City of Hobart in updating their website to include information on how to compost food waste at home. We worked with forty-one households, providing them with free training and support. After just one month, these households had diverted just under 1.5 tonnes of food waste from landfill, reducing greenhouse gas emissions and producing nutrient-dense compost for food production.

The My Smart Garden program in Melbourne's west is a free sustainable gardening behaviour-change program run by Kat Lavers for Hobsons Bay City Council. It helps residents adapt to a changing climate and resource scarcity by turning their outdoors into productive food gardens. The program takes a holistic approach across five elements of sustainable gardening including food production,

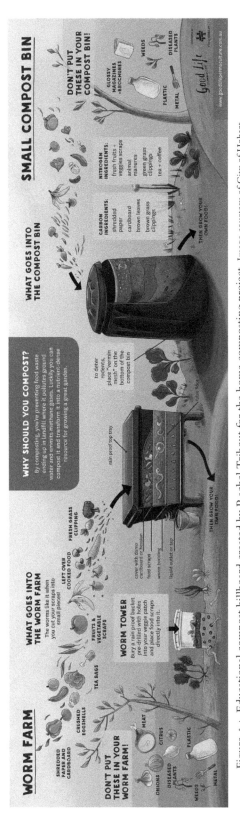

Figure 5.4. Educational compost billboard created by Rachel Tribout for the home composting project. Image courtesy of City of Hobart.

sheltering homes from sun and wind, onsite use of green waste and grey water, and encouraging biodiversity. In 2015, the program was estimated to have helped participants divert at least 51 tonnes of organic waste from landfill, reduce greenhouse gas emissions by 87 tonnes and save at least 2574 kilolitres of potable water! Anecdotal evidence suggests, however, that greatest impact has been seen in the connections between neighbours that have flourished over the shared passion for growing food.

Resilient food systems of the future

Suburban gardens will never be able to grow all our food – we'll always need our rural farmers. In our vision of a resilient food system, perishable foods like herbs, fruits and vegetables are produced locally in people's homes, community spaces and in small urban farms and peri-urban market gardens. Other food enterprises like honey, mushrooms and aquaculture occupy spaces unsuitable for growing, including disused petrol stations and car parks. Some high protein foods such as eggs, dairy (from goats), nuts and meat from small livestock are 'farmed' within the city where appropriate, but are mostly supplied through strong ties with peri-urban farmers. Rural farms produce oil, pulses and grains. Together, the city and country folk provide a complete diet, adapted to our climate and bioregion. There is plenty of evidence that growing food at home makes gardeners more likely to care where their food comes from and, so, another important way that home food gardens contribute to sustainable and resilient food systems is by fostering support for small-scale farmers, both within and beyond the city limits.

Our experience has proven that despite barriers, in particular the lack of skills, the humble home garden has much to offer urban food systems. In the words of William Gibson, 'the future is here, it's just not evenly distributed', and we are constantly being inspired by new permaculture gardens taking root in the suburbs. As we write, these threads are being woven into a future fabric of local food for flourishing urban communities. While policy changes are needed to support access to affordable housing and land, and we must continue to advocate for a fair, sustainable food system at a broader scale, at least on the household front, we already have all the solutions we need. So, we invite you to join us – put your boots on, get outside and begin!

Chapter 6

The Food Forest: Demonstrating a Sustainable Food Production System for Adelaide, South Australia

Graham and Annemarie Brookman

The point of this case study is to demonstrate that commercial quantities of natural, high-quality food can be grown efficiently in urban and peri-urban areas without inconvenience, danger or complaint from neighbours and with significant advantage to the food security, biodiversity and aesthetics of the city.

The idea of building a sustainable farm and learning centre slipped into the minds of Annemarie and Graham Brookman as a result of reading the small book *Permaculture One* by Bill Mollison and David Holmgren. It was the early 1980s and they had already bought a vacant 29-acre piece of land in a northern Adelaide suburb and planted biodiverse windbreaks, but, despite their formal agricultural training and five years of world travel, they had no framework within which to create the polycultural and sustainable farm they dreamed of until permaculture design dropped into their lap. In 1983 they attended a design course with Bill Mollison and within a few weeks had documented a design that is now the Food Forest: a 49-acre farm and learning centre that provides Adelaideans with 150 varieties of certified-organic food, wine, cider and vinegar, employs five local people, sequesters 300 tonnes of CO_2 annually (in increased soil carbon) and welcomes interns from around the world to experience sustainable design in action (see figure 6.1, colour insert). It essentially runs on stormwater and the city's composted green waste and delivers largely unpackaged food to urbanites via the Adelaide Farmers Market. Neighbours are proud of it and the local council supports it in the care of the river corridor and other projects.

Having won awards as one of Australia's top certified organic properties and prime exemplars of Landcare, environmental education and sustainable business as well as one of the best medium-scale permaculture properties in temperate Australia, it is a truly 'complete' permaculture design with management of water, food, shelter and energy combining seamlessly with community care and land-use planning. The enterprise offers courses on sustainable design, self-reliance skills and building, educates school and uni groups, and conducts human-scale research and development. It is the state's focal point for education and networking on straw-bale construction and permaculture. Many thousands of people have visited the Food Forest through its regular open days, events and through its online presence via the web and YouTube channel.

Beginnings

The farm was bought using conventional bank finance, with the couple sinking earnings from their TAFE and uni jobs into buying land and infrastructure to create the venture. Forming a partnership together and getting primary producer status proved to be an efficient business structure.

Agreeing on a business name and mission statement brought social and ethical aims into play, and the key goals emerged as:
- demonstrating that land can be managed in an environmentally sustainable way, producing healthy food and a healthy income;
- sharing information and skills for land management, self-reliance, conservation and food production with others; and
- existing as a rich and beautiful place to live, work and raise children with balance, wisdom and skills.

'Food Forest' was a term Mollison used to describe planned, multi-storey, food-bearing orchards and forests, where a huge percentage of available light is absorbed by the trees, shrubs and herbs, and it resonated with Graham, who had spent time at forest villages in tropical jungles whilst an army medic. He hoped he could create an Australian version, but knew it would be tricky to do justice to the name in the driest state in the world's driest inhabited continent. Offsetting the under 400 millimetres of annual rainfall was a seasonal river that ran (in some winters) along the property's northern boundary. Towering red gums along its course indicated that even when its bed was dry, the river was influencing the groundwater.

Permaculture design invites you to look around the globe at latitudes and altitudes similar to your own when establishing a palette of productive plants. For the Food Forest, drought-hardy species like carob, pistachio, pomegranate, jojoba, olive, fig and grape clamoured for space; pistachios getting the biggest nod with their 30-metre-deep roots. Species were also planted for timber, like Canary Island pines and oaks, as well as Australia's eucalypts for fuel-wood. Wildcards like jujubes, nut pines and field crops like wheat and barley also got the drought-hardiness nod.

Biodiversity is associated with stable systems so a 'biodiversity balance tank' (several hectares of reveg scrub) was planted in the centre of the property and linked to the river corridor by native windbreaks. The insects and birds attracted to it counter pest outbreaks in the orchards and gardens.

Moving onto the land: Shelter and self sufficiency
In 1987, adjacent land was added to the original block, which swung the focus to reimagining and renovating the 1840 homestead. The goal was to achieve energy efficiency and establish a productive vegetable garden and home orchard with the citrus, pomes and stone fruit that had been precluded from the commercial plantings on the original block due to high water requirements. Living on the property allowed the owners to provide the super-productive 'racehorse' species the extra care they needed. Food self-reliance was achieved very quickly and water from the roofs of buildings was captured for domestic use.

Water

Re-focusing on the concept of a food forest, as distinct from a 'food savannah' or 'food desert', the Brookmans pumped irrigation water from the river, but dams were subject to 2 metres of evaporation annually and river flows were extremely erratic and often salty. State (mains) water was an essential backup in summer, but was environmentally expensive as most had been pumped over the Mount Lofty Ranges to Adelaide from the Murray River. In 2001 the Murray ceased flowing into the sea for around two years and the government raised mains water prices and halved the amount irrigators could use, slashing the viability of the property.

A bore was drilled to 60 metres and groundwater from the Q_4 aquifer was used for irrigation. This enabled continued production, but with more local bores withdrawing water from the Q_4, over time it became steadily more saline; despite the government regulation of the aquifer, its usage was clearly unsustainable.

Bill Mollison's advice to 'store water underground' continued to ring in Graham's ears and he heard that the nearby Salisbury Council was purifying stormwater using reedbeds and injecting it into deep aquifers during winter, which could be retrieved for irrigation of public ovals and gardens in summer. This established a sustainable water system largely powered by solar energy. With professional advice, such a system has been created at the Food Forest to withdraw low salinity stormwater from the river and local drains when rapidly flowing and store it in the Q_4 under the farm for summer drip irrigation.

The extraordinary work of Ayappa Masagi in restoring groundwater supplies in India (read his book *Bhageeratha*) also provided inspiration for a quick and effective recharge of the water used by trees from the shallow aquifer. Settled stormwater is pumped into a pit in the centre of the property, from which it gravitates through a simple filter atop a vertical 2.4-metre concrete pipe into the sandy, unconfined aquifer.

Responding to climate change

Despite the success of aquifer recharge, the farm is moving away from apples and nashis to a palette of more drought- and salt-hardy plants, such as pomegranates and jujubes. It has also retained more than half its area for non-irrigated cropping, pasture and agroforestry. This is

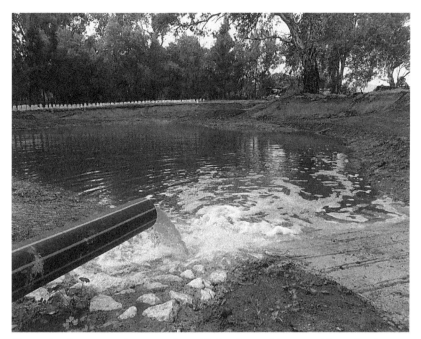

Figure 6.2. Stormwater is captured, purified and stored in an aquifer under the Food Forest for summer irrigation. Photo courtesy of Graham Brookman.

in response to the currently uncontrollable changes caused by global warming, which is

- rapidly reducing the winter chill necessary for many fruit and nut varieties;
- causing extreme heat events;
- reducing rainfall and thus freshwater storage; and
- spectacularly reducing natural aquifer recharge.

Whilst deficit and drip irrigation, mulching and choice of crops and cultivars provide a response to global warming, the increasing intensity of radiation causes outright burning of fruit and nuts. A trial in using sunscreen for plants, made from finely ground limestone, was carried out in collaboration with the organic certifying body National Association for Sustainable Agriculture, Australia (NASAA). Spraying this material onto trees before extreme temperatures (up to 47-degrees Celsius at the Food Forest) has been successful as a transition measure.

Carbon and soil nutrition

Storing more water in the soil can increase moisture infiltration and holding capacity by 100 per cent, delivering a 20 per cent saving in irrigation required. It can increase root mass, biological activity and cation-exchange capacity and decrease root disease, thus increasing yields by 100 per cent. The goal of lifting the farm's soil carbon from a miserable 0.7 per cent to at least 4 per cent seemed achievable and the quest began by spreading 'biosolids' from Adelaide's major sewage plant in 1985. It was a stinky product with suspect quantities of contaminants and it blocked machinery; it was ultimately discarded with the advent of certified organic compost made from waste food and green materials plus some animal manure. It is weed-seed free, free-flowing, contains all the nutrients required for plant growth and includes masses of carbon. Extra carbon came from burning heaps of intractable and thorny pest plants (much of it from along the river) and the mixture of charcoal and ash provided a mineral-rich fertiliser.

Building humus involves countless ubiquitous microbes, but nitrogen fixers were consciously added and a high population of beneficial fungi was encouraged by turning mulch-mowed prunings into the soil before planting crops and pastures. A range of sub-clovers and medics hosted bacteria that fix much of the nitrogen required by crops, and some trees (like carob, casuarina and tagasaste) also associate with Rhizobia and Azotobacter.

The alluvial silt soil of the Food Forest naturally concreted in summer and became a quagmire in winter, so natural gypsum (calcium sulphate) was applied in the early years as a fertiliser and soil conditioner. The calcium ions displace sodium from the colloids making soil more friable. There is occasionally a role for more-manufactured fertilisers, such as abattoir- and fish-processing waste, when strategic applications of high-nitrogen nutrients can make a big difference; for example, helping pistachio trees hold leaves around nut bunches as the filling kernels drag nitrogen from the tree.

Animals

Permaculture design calls for the conservation of energy in all its forms, which encourages the use of as many elements as are feasible in the degradation of an energy source. Plants can be thought of as at the top of the chain, providing energy for humans, animals, fish, invertebrates, fungi and other microbes. The more linkages and the less subsidiary inputs, the more sustainable the process. The Food Forest has particularly included chickens (for eggs, meat, manure, pest control, waste utilisation), geese (for live sale, meat, grass control, manure), sheep (for live sale, meat, broad-leaf plant control, manure) and bettongs (for live sale, pest plant control, revegetation activity). Almost 100 other bird and animal species also inhabit the farm and river corridor. A student map (figure 6.3) of the linkages between elements in the design gives a different picture from an aerial photo and a vital insight into the property's permaculture design, which maximises the number of nutrient and energy flows between its elements, thus using external inputs efficiently and absorbing solar energy, nitrogen gas, rain and flood water, for minimal environmental cost.

Market Garden

Annemarie and Graham had been growing vegetables since they were children and there seemed to be plenty of demand, as they were constantly asked if they could supply neighbours, so launching a market

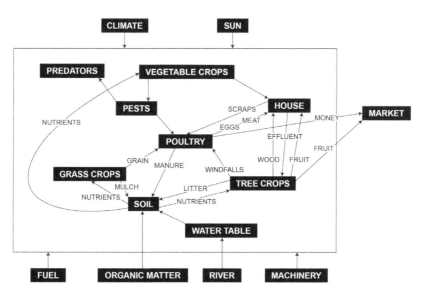

Figure 6.3. A map of the links between elements in permaculture design. Graphic by Kath Chapman, based on Food Forest field trip student report, c. 2010.

garden seemed to be a matter of upscaling their domestic garden. But when a spiritual community of thirty and Adelaide's largest organic veg retailer asked for regular supplies, mechanisation, labour and inputs reared their head – and the question of whether there was a desire to be professional vegetable growers! They limited the area to 1000 square metres. The farm had bought a compact, 60HP orchard tractor, second-hand Agrowplow and offset discs, so creating the first seedbed was deceptively quick.

Graham and Annemarie soon learned why they had success in making mud bricks from the clay silt! Gypsum helped to loosen the soil initially and over time the soil became more resilient as carbon levels topped 10 per cent, but getting the moisture level just right for cultivation is still a critical skill. Two ingredients that made bed preparation a pleasure were the mulching mower, which reduces old sweetcorn plants to a mulch layer of 4 centimetres, and chickens that scratch up weeds and eat their seeds. Compost for the vegies is made from the autumn by-products from processing grapes, pistachios and so on, and a clean out of the chicken run. Soil tests over decades have shown balanced nutrient levels. The dripper tape laterals are numbered for the recording of planting, husbandry and harvest dates, but very little happens apart from a bit of weeding. Wheaten straw mulch suppresses weeds and cools the soil during summer, and the luxuriant growth of winter vegies largely out-competes weeds. To minimise frost damage, no mulch is used in winter. Biodiversity takes care of insect pests and any varieties that exhibit disease susceptibility are discontinued.

Tree crops

Long-term tree crops were planted early in the development of the farm because of their hardiness and relative cheapness since the Brookmans could propagate them. They comprised a wide range of natives, Canary pines and oaks, and a salt-tolerant river red gum variety, Albacutya. Once the trees were recognisable as such, beneficial birds moved in and cleaned up the insect pests like spitfires *(Perga affinis)*. Unlike Norwegian farmers with whom Graham had worked, he did not plant trees as building material for his great grandchildren; he was keen to personally witness both the forestry and agroforestry plantings hard at work, with sheep feeding on acorns, carobs and honey locust pods in shaded comfort and pines being felled to give sawlogs and to give the more permanent oak plantings more space and light. Without enough rain to grow *Pinus radiata, P. canariensis* was an ideal species: slower growing but producing fine-grained reddish timber and fabulous cones for fire-lighting.

The fruit and nut orchards are mainly based on 6-metre inter-row and 5-metre tree spacings, allowing trees plenty of root/soil volume to attain 'normal' size and shape, with good airflow and solar access. They are dressed with approximately 22 cubic metres of 'cultured compost' per hectare annually (Adelaide's green and food waste). It is principally thrown under the tree rather than in the inter-row and performs a mulching role as well as nutrition and soil carbon. Drip irrigation is applied at 3 megalitres per hectare per annum. No machine pruning or harvesting is used in favour of plant health and local employment. Disease control is generally via strategic copper (cuprous oxide) sprays, good training and hygiene combined with variety selection. Weed control is the main husbandry work: geese have been effective as grass-selective mowers, but they left the inter-row dominated by broad-leafed plants, so sheep were introduced to balance the grazing

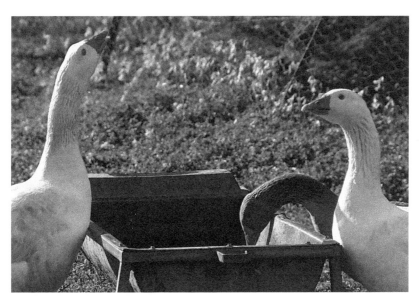

Figure 6.4. Geese are key weed controllers on organic properties. Photo courtesy of Graham Brookman.

and to remove suckers of rootstocks. Conventional Australian breeds were found to damage trees and they require shearing, crutching and so on, so the Food Forest is venturing into breeding a genetically robust mini sheep that sheds its wool in summer.

Value-adding and certification

Annemarie had been wary of agricultural chemicals since a spray-drift incident in her childhood in Holland, so the vegetable garden was managed organically from day one, but the move to certification for the whole property came when a major buyer decided to stock only certified fruit and veg. Annemarie increased the pressure on Graham to convert the orchards and paddocks, and he worked out that he could eliminate herbicide use by introducing geese as selective grazers that would control creeping weeds like couch and kikuyu. A 1.8-metre-high electric fence was erected around the bulk of the property to protect geese, chickens and bettongs from foxes and cats. This system enabled full certification, which conferred price premia of 20 per cent to 100 per cent for products and opened up a market that has grown steadily at over 15 per cent each year.

In the 1990s, the pistachio crop hit volumes that required cold storage at 1 degree celsius, so a straw-bale cold room, with drop-in fridge unit, was erected. It was extremely efficient and could be set at different temperatures, depending on the produce to be held. The nuts still needed to be taken long distances for de-hulling, drying and grading (of the naturally split nuts from the non-splits that frustrate pistachio eaters), and there was a significant cost in transport and certifying the remote plants for the few hours it took to process the crop.

'Why not set up a certified organic, village-scale processing system that we and other local growers could use?', thought the Brookmans. They purchased a second-hand de-hulling system and commissioned a unique electric dehydrator that would dry fruit and herbs as well as nuts. A compact grading machine was ordered from Greece and a cracker to extract the kernels from non-split nuts came from Sicily. An added nut dryer increased throughput by 200 per cent and now other growers are able to bring their nuts and participate in the processing.

A tiny vineyard was established in the '90s and Graham made small batches of wine for domestic consumption. With a few prizes from the local Gawler Wine Show under his belt, he bought a tiny Italian grape and apple crusher and a cheap but extremely effective little filter/bottler, and was introduced to variable volume stainless steel cylinders; he set up a mini winery for a few hundred dollars! His love affair with winemaking has seen the grafting of vines to some of the vine varieties best prepared for climate change and the use of yeasts that flourish under local vineyard conditions. Discovering that he was allergic to sulphur, he manages the vines without it (there are alternatives like copper, whey, milk, potassium bicarbonate, and compost tea). He keeps preservative use in the wine to a bare minimum (maximum forty parts per million sulphur dioxide) and is still producing fruit-driven, long-keeping wines that he and a substantial slab of the population with a sensitivity to sulphur can drink without ill effects.

Marketing

By the 2000s, they needed a better way to market the farm's products than taking small orders to diverse retailers and restaurants, so they approached the Royal Agriculture and Horticultural Society for support to open a farmers market at the Adelaide Showground. Run by a not-for-profit association, it has been a resounding success, with the market attracting 120 stalls and 5000 to 6000 shoppers each Sunday and scoring back-to-back wins as Australia's best farmers market. Most Food Forest product is moved through the Showground market; however, some select retailers are still serviced. The pistachios are distributed by food cooperatives around Australia.

Building and waste systems

Much of our impact on the planet is through the energy required to construct and maintain comfort within our buildings, so the Food Forest formed collaborations with well-known architects and builders of sustainable buildings, particularly using the by-product of cereal growing, straw! It became the medium of choice for the learning centre, cold room, wine cellar, accommodation and garden structures. It was one of the original properties to open for Australia's Sustainable House Day, which can claim significant credit for South Australia's high uptake of passive and active solar home design.

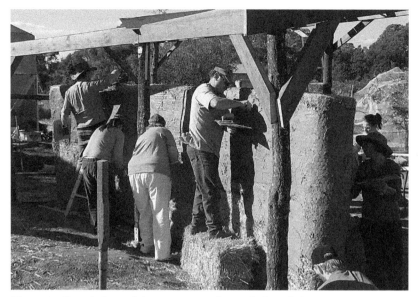

Figure 6.5. Strawbale workshop – constructing an indoor shelter. Photo courtesy of Graham Brookman.

Permaculture design's call to 'create no waste' led to the Food Forest's modern composting toilet and reedbed systems, which have been used as exemplars by organisations and individuals, including local government and the state health department.

Education

As trained teachers, Annemarie and Graham naturally wanted to share their growing knowledge of sustainable living and its underpinning design principles. Responding to the call of permaculture's second ethic, 'Care for community', they opened their home and farm for field-walks and inspections, sharing failures and successes with the public. The demand for information was insatiable, so they offered weekend workshops on organic vegetable growing, fruit production, sustainable building design, straw-bale construction, food preservation, composting toilet and reed-bed systems. Eventually, they teamed up with David Holmgren to offer full permaculture design certificate courses and a suite of fully accredited graduate programs in permaculture through Central Queensland University. All three of Adelaide's universities and many TAFE colleges have used the

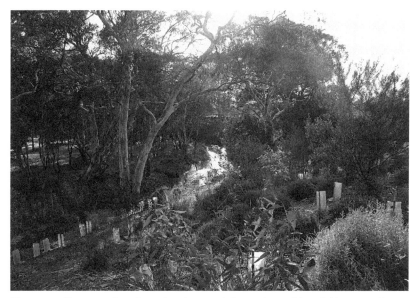

Figure 6.6. Revegetation along the river – a joint project with neighbours and government. Photo courtesy of Graham Brookman.

Food Forest for field visits and lectures in disciplines as varied as agriculture, architecture, environmental management, valuation and hydrogeology.

All this activity could have left children out of the mix, so a school tours program was introduced, giving thousands of kids the chance to see the potential for them to build their own patches of paradise.

Having benefited from working on European and North American farms, Graham was heavily involved in Australia's main exchange program for young agriculturists. He and Annemarie have hosted scores of young people hungering to learn about sustainable land use and, needless to say, the Brookman children have friends scattered across the planet and have both studied and travelled extensively overseas.

Graham's encounter with young British filmmaker Sam Collins, who was desperate to satisfy work requirements to get a second Aussie visa, led to a collaboration that produced some thirty mini-videos and two substantial documentaries, which are publicly available on YouTube, and a movie about permaculture and the designing of the Food Forest. These have reached over a million viewers around the world.

The Food Forest continues to flourish, grow and help others to establish sustainable enterprises. It contributes to public and policy discussion at local and national levels.

Permaculture design

The ethics of permaculture are uncontentious: care for the planet, care for community and personal action towards those ends. If one tests every decision one makes against these ethics, it will ultimately alter the way society works and will produce new research and policies in every field of human endeavour (including urban planning, which currently serves to preclude or hinder urban agriculture and facilitates the building of suburbs over the best soils and aquifers).

Many ask, 'But how do I redesign my behaviour/profession/workplace/home to conform with permaculture ethics?' Just use the logical and science-based permaculture design principles explained in hundreds of short courses, books and websites. The ten-day Permaculture Design Certificate can give you a chance to redesign your life, business, campus, farm or home during the course.

Chapter 7

Garden Farming: The Foundation for Agriculturally Productive Cities and Towns

David Holmgren

Australian suburbs can be transformed into productive, resilient and sustainable places to live through garden farming. Growing food right where people live, in back and front yards, has environmental, social and psychological benefits. Garden farming in the household, non-monetary economy is complementary to commercial urban and peri-urban agriculture that, collectively, can be the heart of a resilient bio-regional food system.

For garden farming to reach its full potential, the paving over of land in the older suburbs through house expansion and infill development must be replaced with better utilisation of existing building stock.

The deflation of the Australian property bubble is more likely to precipitate this necessary change than enlightened policy action. However, direct action by householders retrofitting suburbia will be most critical in creating agriculturally abundant, resilient, people-focused suburbs with a higher quality of life.

My book *RetroSuburbia: The Downshifter's Guide to a Resilient Future*,[1] is a manual and a manifesto to assist householders retrofit the built, biological and behavioural fields of the non-monetary home economy; a process that can start without the permission, support or funding of governments, corporations or banks.

Potential for garden farming Australian suburbs

Garden farming, as well as commercial urban and peri-urban agriculture, is critical to the retrosuburban way of life. I use the term 'garden farming' for small-scale intensive production systems associated with homes and providing primarily for household needs, with human labour rather than machines providing the major power input. This is distinct from commercial food production that is primarily for sale in the monetary economy.

Private open space on residential lots is ideal for intensive garden farming to provide some or all of the household's fresh food, including small livestock products (see figure 7.1, colour insert). This food production in the non-monetary economy is more efficient than the centralised food supply systems, has many environmental benefits, including radically reduced food miles and greenhouse gas emissions, and can be developed without the need for finance, regulation or markets.

There are a wide range of practical and psychological factors that give the growing of food in suburban households great potential.

- Urban areas produce large amounts of organic material, through both food wastage and the management of gardens and other spaces. This can become a critical resource for improving and maintaining soil fertility.
- Reasonably priced, clean water is readily available at pressure in urban areas and the excess of stormwater running off the many hard urban surfaces provides a valuable, but so far under-utilised, resource for garden farming. There is also further potential for recycling greywater[2] as well as the nutrients in humanure[3] through simple and safe composting systems.
- The majority of most Australian suburban landscapes are in benign climates allowing year-round food production. The high levels of sunshine in Australia partly compensate for effects of shading by trees and buildings in urban areas.

- As well as building household resilience, garden farming is a practical and satisfying way to connect with nature. It can accommodate and enhance other outdoor household activities to create a healthier lifestyle that directly addresses the obesity crisis.

Furthermore, extensive adoption of efficient garden farming methods across the suburbs would also help conserve our best arable farmland for growing staple crops and increase society-wide resilience to centralised supply shocks.

It would also help restart the household and community non-monetary economies of gift, barter and reciprocity that have been eroded in recent decades with the credit-fuelled growth in GDP. History shows that any substantial downturn in the monetary economy, especially due to a credit freeze, reboots household self-reliance, as everyone saves scarce money for the things they cannot do for themselves. In such conditions, the fact that householders may not be the most expert food growers or that their sites are less than optimal for garden farming, does not prevent people from growing what they can.

Without foresight by society, the pain and suffering from any economic-, geopolitical-, energy- or climate-induced shocks will be greater than necessary. On the other hand, such shocks might also encourage the most competent garden farmers to go commercial. While small-scale, and even backyard, commercial producers currently supply high-end, boutique urban consumers, under changed conditions they may be part of an expansion of urban agriculture that, in combination with garden farming and bioregional supply chains, could create a parallel food system to the centralised one. This parallel food system is described in my essay, 'Feeding Retrosuburbia: From the Backyard to the Bioregion'.[4] In this way, retrosuburbia could be the nursery or incubator raising a new generation of farmers working at urban, peri-urban and rural scales.

As well as focusing on food production in the household, retrosuburbia involves making full use of, and creatively repurposing, our existing buildings. The last half century's rise in residential property prices[5] has fuelled the building and paving over of water- and carbon-absorbing land needed to feed ourselves into the future and, in the process, is condemning our children to live disconnected from nature, which we depend on for our daily life and wellbeing. Curbing this maddening, frenzied rush involves making better use of the buildings we have to increase population density, whilst allowing both medium-to-large front and backyards and peri-urban fringes to remain available for food production.

My retrosuburbia model is based on the lived reality of a growing number of ordinary Australians who have been influenced by the permaculture concept – a vital emerging global movement that first took root in the suburbs of Australia forty years ago. The impact of permaculture, and the UK spin off, the Transition Towns movement,[6] is at the progressive edge of communities building resilience in a climate-changed world. The Permablitz model that continues to empower young people to change their habitats for the better has also spread around the world from Melbourne.[7]

Such households are already proving the potential of garden farming. Documented examples include:[8]

- one small household producing over 350 kilograms of food annually (and increasing each year) on a 271-square-metre block in inner Melbourne;
- a diverse garden of only 64 square metres with an annual production of more than 234 kilograms of fruit, nuts and vegetables; and
- a small block in Seymour, central Victoria, producing 257 kilograms of vegetables, 163 kilograms of fruit and sixty-five-dozen eggs in one year.

If these yields were being generated with high inputs of energy, chemicals and complex equipment and infrastructure, or required complex processing and distribution chains with high levels of waste and inefficiency (as happens in the centralised supply system), then they would not be so potent in terms of climate change or the wider sustainability debate. Although the study of the environmental and resource conservation benefits of garden farming has barely begun, it is obvious to those with a modicum of understanding of 'life cycle analysis' and other techniques that fresh-food production within the household economy has huge inherent efficiencies compared to the centralised system, even if the kilograms per square metre of commercially acceptable yields are much less than the figures above.

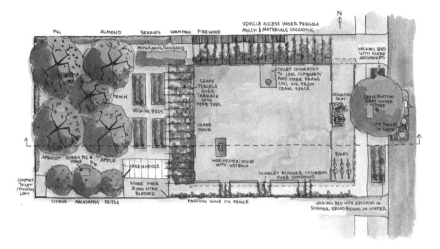

Figure 7.2. Small urban house and garden plan. Image courtesy of Holmgren Design.

The benefits of home food production extend beyond the growing of food. A back-of-the-envelope assessment of fruit bottling at our home property of Melliodora used data from an extensive study of best practice within the centralised food system.[9] It suggested greenhouse gas emissions were about 10 per cent of that of the centralised system due to the permaculture-designed garden farming, micro food miles, repurposed bottles, no packaging, carbon-neutral wood heating for pasteurisation and multitasking, home-based labour.

A retrosuburban diet

In the essay 'Feeding Retrosuburbia: From the Backyard to the Bioregion',[10] I suggested a large minority of Australians living in agriculturally productive retrosuburbia could be getting half their food from a combination of household-level garden agriculture and commercial urban agriculture, with the bulk of the remainder coming from commercial farming within the bioregion. The retrosuburban diet (in the sense of a statistical average rather than a prescription) would involve much higher consumption of vegetables and a lower consumption of meat and dairy, with a significant proportion of the dairy being from goats rather than cows. However, the growth of this bioregional food system to feed the whole population of our largest cities would be unlikely in anything other than more severe future scenarios.

Historical turning point

If my reading of the forces at work in the environment, economy and culture are correct, there is an historic opportunity for the retrosuburban agenda to address numerous stresses felt by Australian households. These range from mortgage stress and energy costs, through health and wellbeing concerns, to avoiding the digital vortex for children.

The interest in food growing at home and backyard poultry, bees and even goats, is now exceeding the wave of interest in the 1970s, while the internet and social media are allowing dispersed networks of interest to share knowledge and support in what Rob Hopkins of the Transition Towns movement has called 'The Great Reskilling'.[11]

The motivations for this self-reliance and downshifting are changing from a focus on values and ethics to encompass a rational economic advantage over lifestyles of high debt, long working hours and high consumption. The credit-fuelled bubble economy of affluent Australia is generating discarded goods, materials and even food at ever increasing rates. This material is being gathered, used and repurposed by a growing cohort of urban and suburban dwellers learning how to live well while consuming much less.

More people sharing houses and spending more time at home promises to revitalise households whilst creating a critical mass of active and present residents in suburbia. This, in turn, increases efficiency in use of costly infrastructure, reduces crime through casual surveillance and builds community connections. It also provides the economies of scale for efficient garden farming and a host of other self-reliance activities that are marginal in one- and two-person households. Larger households are already forming in a variety of ways including extended family consolidation, blended families and various forms of sharing and landlord/tenant arrangements.

The bursting of the current housing bubble in Australia, geo-political stress, energy price shocks and climate-change-induced natural disasters could each trigger a psychosocial and political crisis in affluent and unprepared Australia. There is no doubt that any of these forces would lead to a massive surge in households sharing, reskilling and downshifting to secure their future.

My *RetroSuburbia* book and strategy is positioned to feed the interest in household food production and resilience, but I know it will be the influences of the global economy, superpower competition, resource depletion, and climate and environmental forces – as well as wildcards – that will ultimately be the strongest factors in determining whether the current momentum is sustained or whether it subsides.

Threats and risks

The corporations that dominate the fresh food distribution and retail trade need population growth – and minimal market loss to farmers markets, community-supported agriculture and garden farming – for continued growth. Even a small leakage of customers from the centralised food system is a serious problem for corporations that must grow to keep shareholders happy.

Another set of powerful interests see garden farming as a biosecurity threat to large-scale horticultural and livestock industries. Biosecurity crisis plans could see mass culls of backyard poultry and/or bees, for example, as largely symbolic acts to protect established industries.

One possible version of an energy-descent future that I have coined 'Brown Tech'[12] combines a moderate decline in the availability of high-quality fossil fuels with accelerating climate change. This is likely to trigger a crisis response from central governments with a wide range of natural and geopolitical impacts. The loss of faith in market solutions, acceptance by the majority of a 'command economy' to maintain essential services, including the centralised food system, and a general sense of crisis could see organic, bottom-up solutions marginalised or even suppressed as threats to the centralised systems.

The question before us now is whether the growth in garden farming and urban agriculture, as well as a rebooting of the household and community non-monetary economies in our suburbs, goes viral or whether it retreats to enclaves in the shadows of an increasingly armoured and centralised economy.

Countering infill development

Powerful interests will continue to target the Australian suburban heartlands as the place for increasing infill development, which builds and paves over critical territory for garden and urban farming.

Governments have historically relied on immigration to drive growth in GDP, and regular efforts to convince Australians, especially in Melbourne and Sydney, to accept the need to infill the suburbs are increasing. The bursting of the property bubble could leave governments with very few options to maintain growth in the monetary economy.[13]

Ironically, environmental and social-equity arguments are used to justify infill as the best option for responding to the growth in population in our capital cities and regional towns.[14] Even accepting the flawed argument that great population density is essential for our suburbs to be sustainable, four decades of incremental infill development has failed to increase population density.[15] Despite this complete failure, infill proponents call for an acceleration to cover the middle belt of suburbs in our capital cities with apartments, which would destroy their garden farming potential.

The entrenched interests of Australia's largest industry – property development and construction – combined with myopia, lack of rigor in academia and politics, and a mostly disempowered public have seen this debate intensify. However, the discussion of real alternatives, in particular those grown from ideas and innovations such as my retrosuburbia strategy, does not form part of this national debate.

The orthodoxy accepted by the majority of planners, academics and even environmentalists that higher population density is the key to improved urban amenity, viable public transport, infrastructure efficiency, lower environmental impact and even resilience to climate change is built on many other flawed assumptions including that:

- economic growth is an unquestioned good that will continue into the future more or less perpetually;
- the elimination of soil, plant and animal life in favour of more building is collateral damage that can be compensated for by token symbols of our ongoing metabolic and psychosocial dependence on nature;
- the daily movement of the majority of residents beyond walking or even cycling distances is an essential element of urban life;
- the just-in-time movement and on-demand availability of food and all the other essentials of life to this constantly moving population is necessary and sustainable into the future, and

- the provision of our needs within the household and community non-monetary economies is an unnecessary remnant of the past that can be replaced by new forms of consumerism in the monetary economy.

The truth of the matter is this: we do not have a lack of buildings to house people. At the 2016 census there were over one million vacant dwellings, 200,000 more than a decade ago.[16] There are endless rooms, garages, sheds and other spaces full of stuff no one has time to use. By forming larger households of extended family or likeminded people, taking in boarders and leasing spare spaces, as well as retrofits to other buildings, we can eliminate the need for more large-scale re-developments that threaten suburban food-growing potential. At the same time, we can begin to make some inroads into the triple and linked crises of homelessness, housing affordability and social isolation that lead to loneliness and mental health conditions.[17]

There is a risk that those committed to protecting critically important peri-urban agricultural land could become convinced to support infill development as a way to avoid urban sprawl. In this way, the environment movement could be split because of a lack of imagination and rigour in the urban sustainability debate.

Incremental and powerful change

In the early years of the permaculture movement, designers and activists took for granted that a permaculture revolution would begin with self, household and communitarian reliance outside the monetary economy. The bigger vision included the transformation of the economic, political and social order through this bottom-up process. For permaculture activists, the descriptor 'revolution disguised as gardening' encapsulated the nascent permaculture movement.

In the years since, the permaculture movement has struggled to be recognised as more than a fashionable form of organic gardening; however, retrosuburbia shows how permaculture thinking can transform agriculture and society in the way that the word suggests.

Recognising, articulating and quantifying garden farming as nurturing the food producers and consumers of future food systems is an important task that academics can support. Better documenting of garden farming case studies will improve the evidence base for policies, but also runs the risk that high profile examples will be targeted for discrediting by powerful interests driving the infill-development agenda. Consequently, defending garden farming in the household and community non-monetary economy could become necessary, which may even re-energise community-level oppositional environmentalism.

To make our cities and suburbs agriculturally abundant and lovable human habitats, advocates, activists and educators should focus on supporting the growing number of household garden farmers to become more effective and productive as the critical pathway to this larger vision.

Chapter 8

Citizen Design, Permaculture and Community-based Urban Agriculture

Morag Gamble

At Northey Street City Farm, established in Brisbane in 1994, we operate the farm on permaculture principles. The farm supports a plant and seedling nursery and a weekly farmers market, as well as running numerous workshops and events. It receives many thousands of visitors every year and is seen as a highlight of a trip to Brisbane. As well as being a founding member of Northey Street City Farm, I have also been extensively involved in the Australian City Farms and Community Gardens Network, as well as the Crystal Waters Permaculture Village, and have run my own permaculture organisation since 1998. I believe that focusing on the re-localisation of our food systems can catalyse a great many positive changes in society, including a reconnection with the land, with our communities and ourselves. In this chapter, I reflect on my twenty-five years of experience in working for sustainable, fair and resilient urban food systems in Brisbane, south east Queensland and beyond.

The story of urban agriculture I share is a community-based one – of communities designing, growing, harvesting, making, sharing, learning and teaching together, as well as helping other

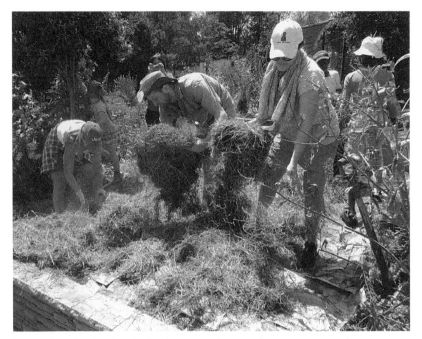

Figure 8.1. The simple art of making a garden together connects people to one another and to place. Photo courtesy of Evan Raymond.

neighbourhoods get started too. It is a story of the emergence of what I call 'citizen designers' and the activation of communities to re-imagine and reclaim the commons for food abundance and positive change – for people and the planet.

You can find communities cultivating local food projects just about everywhere – they create better places to live that are more caring, meaningful and abundant. By growing food together, people can build resilience and improve the liveability of their neighbourhoods, and many positive ripples flow from this.

My involvement with urban agriculture in the commons includes experiences in Australia, UK, Spain, Turkey, USA, Hong Kong, South Korea and Cuba. In response to the increasing call for assistance and information from local communities, I collaborated with others to create the Australian City Farms and Community Gardens Network, which set out to help and support this movement in Australia.

Since the early 1990s, I've been involved in a wide variety of urban agriculture projects in public parks, universities, schools and

community centres. I have observed that the most flourishing and resilient community-based urban agriculture projects do a number of things. They:
- connect people to each other, to food and to place.
- nurture belonging and shared responsibility. People who feel engaged are happier and give more of their time, energy and resources to that shared project.
- learn and share together. The wealth of knowledge, skills and experience in a neighbourhood is vast.
- revitalise a sense of the commons, demonstrating new ways of relating to and using the shared spaces in our cities rather than being passive consumers of public space.
- create a food lens to see our neighbourhoods' thriving food potential.
- tell a new food story, changing the image we have in our minds of what a food garden looks like and the story we tell ourselves about where our food comes from.
- help people see beyond the boundaries and care what is happening to the quality of their local environment, including the state of their waterways, how polluted things are, how much litter is lying around and the quality of habitat for other species.
- regularly celebrate successes and show gratitude to each other, to supporters, mentors and to the earth.
- engage and cultivate citizen designers.

Citizen design

I want to talk more about citizen design because it is a new concept in the realm of urban agriculture. Without a doubt, the most robust and resilient urban community gardens and city farms I have seen in many parts of the world have active, happy groups that typically employ what I call citizen design processes focused on being community-based, participatory, collaborative and connecting. These groups are concerned with the *way* they do things, in addition to their practical goals, and are conscious of reflecting on and refining their people processes regularly.

I describe 'citizen design' as the process involved in cultivating the practical skills, commitment and civic enthusiasm that people need in order to be actively involved in creating a vision, designing, building and caring for the commons. It's about creating great local places that respond to the neighbourhood's needs and reflect its particular character.

I have found permaculture to be a valuable tool for cultivating citizen designers in community-based urban agriculture projects. Permaculture is an accessible, ecological design system that helps people design sustainable human habitats and food abundance within the ethical framework of 'earth care, people care and future care'. Permaculture education strengthens a neighbourhood's capacity to design and create regenerative food projects. Being a worldwide movement, permaculture also connects citizen designers with a global network of design mentors.

The citizen design approach helps more people to be actively involved in community-based urban agriculture projects. This builds resilience because people feel able to create and manage things autonomously within their neighbourhood. They understand how things works, know how to change things, how to fix things and how

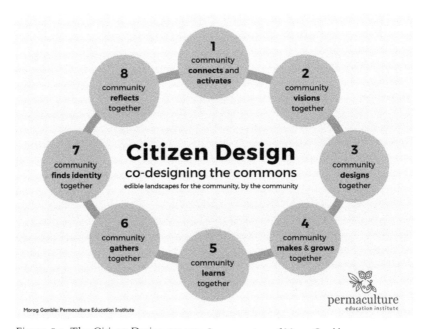

Figure 8.2. The Citizen Design process. Image courtesy of Morag Gamble.

to evolve the project as the community changes and grows. Active participation and knowledge sharing is everything.

After learning more about the idea of citizen science, I realised that how we have been creating community gardens and city farms has actually been a 'citizen design' process – citizens activating and becoming engaged in designing public space for public good. It's not a term I had heard before, but it made such good sense. In community gardens, neighbours come together to have a vision, design, create and benefit from the project.

Collaborative or participatory design processes are of course not new and are often used in community gardens. This type of process-oriented, participatory design emerged in Scandinavia in the 1970s.[1] It is now more commonly known as co-design (cooperative design) – a method typically used in place-making. It describes a process of co-creation and open participatory design.[2] Participatory design, however, usually involves an external motivation and directive.

In defining citizen design in relation to urban agriculture projects in Brisbane, I describe a deeper level of activation and engagement – where the motivation and inspiration comes from within the community and people collaborate to design and implement a project to meet their needs in a flexible and evolving way, seeking support from experts on their own terms. I describe citizen design as 'design by the community, for the community, on common land'.

I went searching for other places where the term 'citizen design' had been used. In New York, the idea of the citizen designer is just emerging. A group of urban designers and architects are asking the question, 'How can the average citizen initiate participation and contribute to the progress of the city?'[3] They recognise that everyone is part of the design process and good design happens when citizens are given the tools and are invited to the design table from the outset.

Citizen design in action: Northey Street City Farm, Brisbane

Northey Street City Farm is an iconic community urban agriculture project established in 1994 in Brisbane. It has been a catalyst for activating the local food scene in Brisbane and is a place of community connection, community education, community action, community visioning, community culture and community economy.

This city farm has inspired the spread of local community gardens, farmers markets and food groups. Not long after we began the city farm, people started asking for help to start community garden projects in their own neighbourhoods, and before long there was a growing network of community gardens around Brisbane.

Although I had been exploring urban agriculture for some years, my real education began with the establishment of this city farm, and many of the lessons I have shared already have been distilled from my experience here.

Northey Street's story is of community-led transformation and place-making through a permaculture and local food lens. It is a tale of how an abandoned and unused park near the centre of Brisbane became a thriving urban food hub that leads, inspires and helps people to live a more sustainable, nature- and community-connected life in the city.

Ritually, thousands flock to Northey Street City Farm each week for a taste of the good life: good food, good music, good conversation, grounding, a peaceful environment, shared gardening, nature play, garden yoga, to learn something new, to meet with people who care, to hang out under the huge mango tree and just soak it all in (see figure 8.3, colour insert). It's more than a food hub, it's a platform for positive change, a thriving human habitat and also now a place where people have created a livelihood that fits with their ethics.

Northey Street City Farm is a great example of citizen design. Right from the very start, there was a clear goal that this educational food forest was being created by the people, for the people, on the commons.

The city farm's thriving gardens have now grown to inhabit 4 hectares of public land only 3 kilometres from downtown Brisbane. The busiest hospital in the city is just across the creek and one of Australia's biggest spaghetti junctions has risen up around it. But even with all this going on, there is an amazing sense of calm as soon as you wander through the edge plantings into heart of the city farm. People (especially kids) so often comment on the sense of being in an oasis, where things are a bit wilder, where time slows down, where people connect, listen, talk, grow food and share meals together. The difference from the normal urban reality is palpable and that is what keeps drawing people back and makes them want to create a piece of this in their own local neighbourhoods.

How did the city farm start?
In 1993, a small group of friends started to dream the city farm into existence. We would meet every week and walk along the river catchment looking for a piece of land. We came from different backgrounds but were united by a desire to grow food together and create an example of sustainable living in the city. Our group was passionate about community, permaculture, organic food, cooperatives, eco-consumerism, social justice and bush care.

In April 1994, after almost a year of exploring possible locations and making friends with council members (a most important step), we received a one-year trial lease of a hectare of parkland on the banks of Breakfast Creek, a tributary of the Brisbane River. Immediately, we invited the surrounding neighbours to shared meals to get to know each other and explore ideas together. We held co-design sessions and began our weekly gardening days to get the food forest and no-dig garden beds started (the ground was too hard to dig!).

Now, more than twenty years later, you can wander through a lush subtropical food forest scattered with allotment gardens, a kitchen garden, wicking beds, chickens, a composting hub, an education centre and office, the edible landscapes nursery, a weekly organic farmers market, an established timber plantation, beehives, a bush foods hedge, significant creek bank restoration areas, an urban backyard demonstration garden, an active community kitchen, a handmade playground, sound garden and a bike path. The list goes on.

When you look at the thriving landscape and activity today, it's hard to believe that it all started as a severely compacted park with no community connection, little shade, no water, no power, no seats, no play spaces, no toilets and very few trees. To support our first plantings, we carried water in buckets on a stick across our shoulders – and without toilets we only gathered for half-day sessions. For a cup of tea, we boiled the billy on a campfire under a big mango tree and rested on old stump seats. Even the Lord Mayor came to share billy tea with us. We loved it – the simple life. It's not surprising that, even now, people still gather under these big mangoes and important discussions about the future of the farm still happen there.

It will be turning twenty-five years old in April 2019 and, in that time, has become a social, cultural and environmental institution in Brisbane. There is just so much community support for and attachment to the place. Recent threats of closure due to the discovery of contaminated soil met with such public outcry that, instead, a solution was negotiated and a soil strategy put in place. Being a public park in a floodplain there are, fortunately, no threats from urban development, so it looks set to continue into the indefinite future.

There are fifteen part-time employees (plus thirty regular volunteers) now involved and it is largely self-funded through its three core enterprises – the organic farmers market, the education programs and the edible landscape nursery. Because the markets have emerged as the core income stream, the farm is now planning to further develop the 'foodie' side of its activities over the next few years with new initiatives such as a local food café, a cooking school and better outdoor venue spaces for events.

Building community trust

One of the first things you notice about the city farm is the absence of fencing. Everyone is welcome anytime. Instead of a fence, we built relationships and connections to include people and cultivate a sense of shared responsibility for the gardens.

While we were getting started, I lived just up the road from the farm and every day I watered the new trees, checked the chickens and chatted with people wandering in the gardens. One day I noticed that our grafted lemon (a newly donated tree) had shrunk. On closer inspection, I realised that someone had actually removed the grafted tree and in its place planted a bush lemon. We were disappointed, of course, but humoured that the tree thief was thoughtful at least.

In the establishment phase of the city farm, we never locked our shade house, but left seedlings and herb cuttings outside that were surplus to our needs. People would take these but we'd often find gifts left outside the nursery for us in return. When we had a glut of produce, we'd leave a basket in the middle of the farm with a sign inviting people to take some home. This approach was strategically done to reduce people just taking anything – and it worked. It built a relationship of mutual trust and respect.

One late afternoon I noticed a few teenage lads hanging about. I knew that the public buildings further along the creek catchment were regularly graffitied and we'd just designed and built our first structure on the farm. It proudly housed the first public compost toilet in Brisbane City. When I first saw the boys, I began to imagine what damage they might do, but immediately realised I had to flip my thinking.

With a surge of courage, I approached them, chatted with them about the place and invited them to decorate the blank wall (which admittedly did look quite dull in the midst of our lovely gardens). I left it at that and walked away hoping I'd done the right thing. The next morning I hesitantly cycled down to the farm but was absolutely overwhelmed by what I found. The boys had taken up my offer and had painted the wall! In the middle was a huge colourful flower surrounded by a swirling of love hearts and in the corner was their little tag. I never saw the guys again to thank them, but we never had a graffiti issue at the farm. A big lesson from this was that we need to give trust first.

The ripple effect

As you can imagine, being involved in a project like this is incredibly empowering. It is not surprising that many spin-off projects have happened as people found their voice, their confidence to act and learnt skills to be engaged, compassionate and active citizens.

I have seen and been part of new community gardens, street gardens, local food buying groups, community cafes and farmers markets. People have connected around social justice issues, community art and music projects, garden-based playgroups, tool sharing, car sharing, bike fix-it clubs and more. Many have become involved in sharing the story through community food advocacy, study circles, permaculture education initiatives, radio, television, film and articles. Others, including me, have launched their careers from the city farm in urban permaculture consulting and education, gardening, food enterprises, plants, event organising and so much more. Northey Street City Farm's story of community activation is very much echoed in the later Transition Town movement.[4]

What the community envisioned and continues to dream about and achieve on this urban site is nothing short of remarkable. It shows so clearly what is possible when a community is enabled and engaged to create spaces that have meaning, that are responsive to their needs and are able to continually evolve to do this. There is a sense of freedom at the farm – a freedom to think, design, contribute and co-create a neighbourhood that reflects the ethics and values of the people who care and earth care. The city farm has cultivated two decades of citizen designers who continue to ripple their positive approach wherever they live and work.

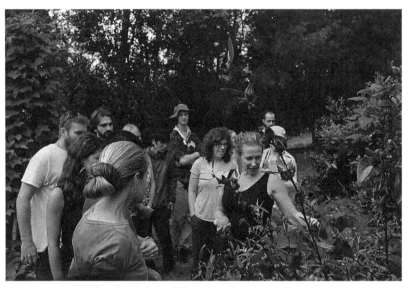

Figure 8.4. So much valuable knowledge about how to read the landscape and grow food sustainably is passed on orally between generations and cultures. Creating opportunities for this exchange to happen is so important. Photo courtesy of Evan Raymond.

PART 3

The New Face of Urban Agriculture in Australia

Chapter 9

Green World Revolution: Urban Farming as Social Enterprise

Toby Whittington and Ali Sumner

Outside a popular bar in the Perth CBD, six of us perched on stools around a high table. With the sun slowly setting behind the city buildings and, after a hectic week supplying fresh produce to thirty-five top restaurants, everyone was happy. It was halfway between Christmas and New Year at the close of 2017. We all clinked our glasses together, celebrating another year at Green World Revolution (GWR).

Three of us had experienced long-term unemployment and one of us had been under-employed before finding employment with GWR. Unlike other, similar enterprises, however, we had founded GWR as a not-for-profit social enterprise in the hope we could help alleviate social and environmental problems with urban farming.

We were relaxed and jolly, each of us reflecting on the year just gone and laughing about our various plans for New Year's Eve. Ali leaned over to Craig and asked him how he was feeling after working with GWR for almost three years. 'Great', he replied. 'It's what I really want to do now and, you know, maybe my son, maybe he's going to grow up and be an urban farmer too.'

When he first came to GWR, Craig didn't know much about plants or woodworking or composting or seasonal veggies and knew nothing about urban farming. He came because he had to undertake a work-for-the-dole activity to continue receiving his unemployment benefit from the Australian Government Department of Social Services. He and his pregnant partner were sharing a low-rent house with aggressive people they didn't like, in a low socio-economic area they didn't want to live in, widely reported in 2013 to have the highest incidence of assaults in the Perth metropolitan area.[1]

As founders of GWR, we are well aware of the reality of Craig's life and the lives of other long-term unemployed people prior to them getting a job working with our organisation. We are familiar with the statistics that in 2016 identified unemployment as one of the highest indicators of poverty in Australia.[2] More significantly, however, by the end of 2017, we had worked with hundreds of long-term unemployed adults at GWR's urban farms. During our weekly welcome 'circle' for new work-for-the-dole participants at our first farm in East Perth, we had heard the same stories over and over: the struggle to find cheap housing, to look after children, to live without a car, to only have a car to live in, to pay an electricity bill, to pay for food or to even have the train fare to travel to our farm to do work for the dole, so a 'bloke can actually get the dole'.

Sitting in the Perth CBD at the end of 2017, a short distance from GWR's second urban farm, we raised our glasses as founders to our first group of long-term employees and handed them each a small gift for helping us grow the farms that would help grow more jobs. It was then, possibly for the first time, we realised GWR was on its way to achieving what we had mused, back in 2012, that it could do, might do and would do.

The ups and downs of starting up

In early 2012, the Western Australian Government established a Social Enterprise Fund with a grants program for not-for-profit organisations. At the same time, Green World Revolution was being established as a not-for-profit company limited by guarantee, to specifically focus on helping solve social problems (such as unemployment) and problems associated with climate change and the degradation of the natural environment. We aimed to do this through urban, suburban and peri-urban horticulture.

GWR was very much in its infancy. We had a founding chief executive officer (Toby), a founding chairperson (Ali) and a small founding board of directors, but no urban farm. Nevertheless, we boldly applied for a grant from the Social Enterprise Fund to establish Perth's first urban farm as a pilot project. This is not to say that Perth had never had city farming activities before GWR came along.

Community gardens and a community farm just outside the Perth CBD had been operating for many years. However, the difference between these activities and GWR's proposed urban farm was the focus on developing the capacity to scale up GWR's operations from one urban farm to many, to grow new jobs while greening urban environments.

Because GWR was specifically founded to deliver positive social and environmental outcomes in a financially sustainable way, unlike other organisations that ran city-based farms or community gardens in Western Australia at the time, GWR was also established, right from the beginning, as a 'social enterprise', as defined by Social Traders (Australia): 'Social Enterprises are driven by a public or community cause, be it social, environmental, cultural or economic. They derive most of their income from trade, not donations or grants, and use the majority (at least 50 per cent) of their profits to work towards their social mission.'[3]

Fortunately, this approach aligned with the Social Enterprise Fund's purpose and by December 2012 GWR had received a grant to establish a pilot urban farm. We were confident we had done our homework, with thorough research of rooftop urban farms, particularly in North America, where urban farming was flourishing. We had consulted with engineers, architects and urban planners and we were ready to start greening the city with urban farming. We enthusiastically re-connected with the property manager who, also with much enthusiasm, had provided 'in-principle' support for GWR's funding application to establish a pilot urban farm on a low-level rooftop annex of one of Perth's tallest CBD buildings.

When the time came to physically set up a pilot farm, the reality of establishing rooftop, city-based farming in Western Australia soon hit home. With the discovery that the area we had been offered was covered in a thick layer of pea gravel, which could not be tampered with because of the waterproof membrane covering the entire area under the gravel, we immediately started looking for an alternative site. It soon became apparent there was no shortage of possibilities and there were many people keen to help – the concept of urban farming on city-based rooftops was de rigeur in 2012, even in Perth. Each time we got to the reality of a site visit, however, it became apparent that establishing an urban farm at a rooftop location in the Perth CBD gave rise to insurmountable challenges. The primary problems were suitable access, after-hours security and, most of all, the almost universal problem of rooftop waterproof membranes that no one wanted damaged or disturbed in any way.

Once we realised that, unlike snow-bearing rooftops in New York, current buildings in Perth – and possibly all Australian cities – are structurally unsuitable for urban farming, we had to challenge all our assumptions about our pilot farm. We abandoned the idea of rooftop farming and started looking for ground-based urban sites devoid of vegetation, only to realise that opposite where our CEO was living (in a commercially zoned area, less than 10 minutes from the Perth CBD) there was a perfect site. Subsequently, we negotiated short-term use of a small piece of land for a 'pop up' farm on the basis GWR would remove 'a bit of stuff' off the site.

A call went out on our newly set up Facebook page. The first weekend we started to build the farm, only four volunteers turned up. A little less help than we had hoped for, but nevertheless we successfully removed 'the bit of stuff', that, in fact, turned out to be 16 cubic metres of building rubble and waste.

Within weeks, in-ground beds had been planted with above-ground planter boxes established and more volunteers kept turning up to help. Enthusiasm was high and a 'community garden' feeling enveloped us all.

Getting down to business

GWR was not established to develop community-garden style activities. We wanted to make a difference to the lives of long-term unemployed people by growing urban farming jobs, while at the same

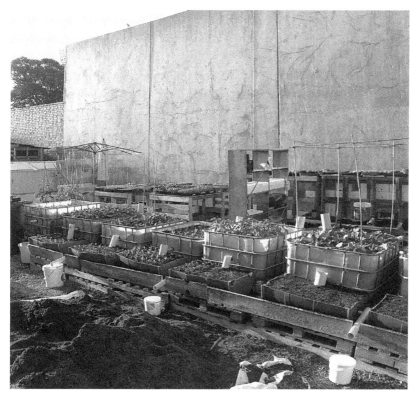

Figure 9.1. Green World Revolution Farm Pilot Site 2013. Photo courtesy of Toby Whittington and Ali Sumner.

time 'greening' urban spaces. We had to move away from volunteer-heavy operations and growing whatever seemed good to eat. We needed to develop a pilot farm that could demonstrate commercial viability. However, with no funds to draw on, other than the rapidly decreasing grant money, we faced a big dilemma. It was like we were trying to find the definitive answer to: what comes first, the chicken or the egg?

Should we be generating sales, when GWR only had a community-garden style operation with some produce, but very little of anything specifically? Or, should we put all our energy into increasing production for commercial supply, while not knowing what was going to sell?

We resolved this dilemma by taking an action-learning approach to everything GWR was attempting to do, an approach that still underpins GWR's operations and will always be inherent in its modus operandi. Basically, adhering to the experiential learning process often referred to as the Kolb Learning Cycle[4] (concrete experience > reflective observation > abstract generalisation > active experimentation > repeat the cycle), GWR decided to specifically focus on testing the hospitality market.

The CEO got out of the farm and onto the road, visiting dozens of restaurants, talking with head chefs and restaurant owners, gaining an understanding of the trends and innovations occurring in the hospitality industry. The response of the chefs was fundamental to building GWR's expertise as an urban farming organisation capable of supplying top-quality produce for Perth's top-quality restaurants.

Integrated within the action learning process focusing on market needs, wants and acceptance with regard to fresh produce was the action learning associated with physically growing this produce in ways that addressed a variety of problems, from Perth's climate and seasonal weather changes to rodents and birds. Then there was the challenge of constantly having to introduce new ways to develop an economically viable supply chain that started with finding reliable seed suppliers, then fine tuning ways to grow produce to meet escalating demand, through to delivering produce to restaurants and cafes on electric bicycles (see figure 9.2, colour insert).

The most significant problem, however, was the cost associated with obtaining urban spaces. GWR had to find a way to be commercially viable on very small pieces of land. GWR's strategic decision to operate many small, commercially viable urban farms in the long-term was therefore driven by the development of GWR's pilot farm, on a 'pocket-size' piece of land, within the first year of our registration as a not-for-profit organisation.

In the summer months of 2013, GWR strengthened its marketing-savvy approach to building sustainable relationships with chefs. Focusing on meeting the needs of Perth's hospitality industry with high-quality niche produce became paramount. We supplied the first micro-herbs in Perth that were not flown in from Melbourne; we responded quickly and grew edible flowers when chefs started asking for them; and we went out of our way to develop climate-appropriate seeding and propagation processes to grow gourmet produce that met the specific needs of Perth's top restaurants. All the while we told our story: 'We are growing urban farms to grow jobs for previously unemployed people. If you help us by buying our produce, you will be helping us to get people out of poverty'.

With the successful completion of the pilot project, by June 2013 we were ready to move off borrowed land and launch our first GWR urban farm. Through persistence and a bit of luck, we successfully secured a long-term lease on a block of land only a few metres down the road from where our pilot project had operated.

One Sunday we moved everything we had established onto a barren, gravel-covered, 400-square-metre space sandwiched between inner-city housing and a warehouse, with a large immovable concrete slab covering at least 150 square metres slap bang in the middle. Our trip down the road also included installing a huge worm farm that we had been given by Murdoch University via a crane suspended from the back of a truck. Having grown our commercial sensitivity, we project-managed the whole move without missing a beat in supplying our increasing list of restaurant clients. We had successfully designed above-ground, totally mobile growing systems during the piloting phase, so they were moved and installed with no break in production or supply. The next day, GWR's Gladstone Street Farm in East Perth was open for business (see figures 9.3a and 9.3b, colour insert).

Our social enterprise challenge

With support from the hospitality industry growing, our list of seasonal products increasing and our ability to produce high-quality produce on time at the right price constantly improving, we turned our attention to being a social enterprise in action, not just in name. More questions had to be answered: What did it mean for GWR to be a social enterprise? What social outcomes did we want to deliver and for whom?

Focusing our attention on these issues, by 2015 we had conceptually developed a GWR pathway-to-employment model for long-term unemployed people to start their involvement with GWR through work-for-the-dole (WFTD) projects. We were very clear as to how we defined ourselves – as a social enterprise – and decided to focus on growing employment opportunities by having direct contact with long-term unemployed people by becoming a WFTD host organisation. We were now running a commercial operation and no longer relied on volunteers to help us at the Gladstone Street farm.

We also began developing an outcomes-based, 'whole-person', adult-learning framework to provide long-term unemployed adults with skill-building and personal development opportunities in how to run an urban farm in a commercial and financially sustainable way. This approach focused on helping WFTD participants take an active role in their own development, meet the requirements of being a member of a group-oriented work environment and make a personal contribution to the betterment of the workplace.

Focusing on helping people to grow feelings of confidence and pride, develop positive attitudes towards themselves as well as others, and learn effective communication, problem solving and creative thinking skills was just as important for GWR as helping them learn the technical and physical skills associated with urban farming.

By the end of 2016, as a WFTD job host working with a large Australian Government–contracted job services provider, we were providing forty places a day for long-term unemployed people to undertake their WFTD obligations for up to six months. We provided work experience, skill building and personal support four days a week at our Gladstone Street farm or at AGWA Botanical, our second urban farm established in liaison with the Western Australian Art Gallery on land at the back of the gallery, closer to the Perth CBD.

By this time, GWR had worked with over 500 WFTD participants and provided paid employment for twenty previously long-term unemployed adults. We had also come to realise that the learning environment we wanted to provide for long-term unemployed people to successfully develop new skills, to become stronger within themselves as well as job-ready for urban farming, was somewhat incompatible with the WFTD system.

Essentially, the growing tension between GWR and the WFTD system centred around GWR focusing primarily on 'outcomes' and the WFTD system focusing primarily on 'outputs'. GWR defines outcomes and outputs in accordance with the internationally accepted definition provided by the W. K. Kellogg Foundation,[5] with *outcomes* being the 'specific changes in behaviour, knowledge, skills…or level of functioning' of people who benefit from the resources that are being allocated. *Outputs*, however, are the 'direct products of the...activities' that are being resourced and 'may include types, levels and targets of services' that are being delivered; for example, the number of people who attend a WFTD project and for how long.

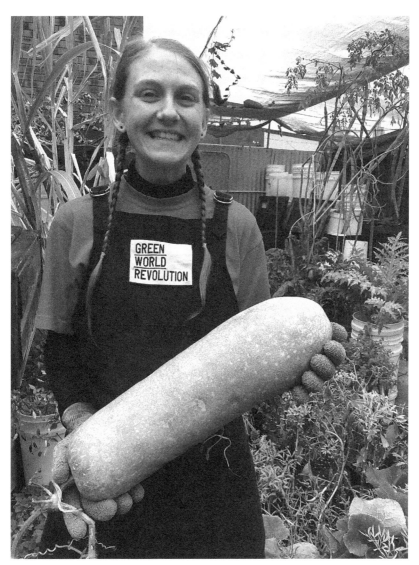

Figure 9.4. Jessica, previously unemployed for two-and-a-half years, harvesting produce at Green World Revolution's Gladstone Street Farm, winter 2018. Photo courtesy of Toby Whittington and Ali Sumner.

Committing to social enterprise urban farming

By the beginning of 2017 it had become obvious that GWR as a social enterprise was obligated to find better ways of maintaining a balance between all its decision-making and actions associated with delivering social value (outcomes not just outputs), environmental value and financial value. We had to start walking our talk more diligently.

Income from delivering WFTD programs was increasing, while income from the sale of produce wasn't. We had fallen into the trap many not-for-profit organisations fall into: over-reliance on project funding with little working capital.

Never afraid of challenging our assumptions, doing things differently, creating new ways and inventing new processes, we suspended our involvement with the WFTD scheme, even though WFTD programs had become our major source of income in 2017. We took a leap of faith and cut what had become our major income source to zero.

As GWR founders, we had always used Dr Edward de Bono's thinking tools, such as the 'Six Thinking Hats®' and authentic 'lateral thinking', as well as 'power of perception' problem solving and decision-making tools, in developing GWR.[6] Also, the GWR board of directors had always used the Six Thinking Hats® for board meetings, with several directors, like the CEO and chairperson, having been trained in the use of these thinking tools. It was a given, therefore, that this arsenal of thinking tools and processes would be applied as we set about developing the next phase of GWR's growth. Our strategic thinking resulted in GWR focusing on four major tasks by the middle of 2017.

Firstly, we needed to re-design and improve GWR's urban farming procedures with a focus on supply chain improvements (including stock ordering, seeding, harvesting, delivery and cutting costs), but not at the expense of quality. Secondly, we looked to diversifying income streams by applying for registration as a charity with the Australian Charities and Not-For-Profit Commission (ACNC) and gaining deductible gift-recipient status with the Australian Taxation Office (ATO). Thirdly, we worked to innovatively design the type of urban farm that could sustainably support the employment of at least three long-term unemployed adults; be commercially viable through the sale of produce to the hospitality industry and consumers; legally function in any local government area in Australia; and incorporate environmentally sound practices in all aspects of its operations.

Fourthly, we wanted to design an innovative social enterprise business model for GWR urban farming that is robust enough to drive the proliferation of GWR-designed urban farms across Australia and fully incorporate skilling, supporting and employing long-term unemployed Australians for the direct relief of poverty.

What next?

By March 2018, GWR had become a registered charity. An innovative social-enterprise business model was being finalised; a new business partnership had been forged to help capitalise our urban farming operations; and our organisation was poised to start proliferating social enterprise urban farms across Australia. Watch this space!

Chapter 10

The Wagtail Urban Farm Story

Steve Hoepfner

'So what are you doing with that block in Mitchell Park?' asked Nat. Nat Wiseman was one of the most knowledgeable growers I'd met in my short farming 'career', so when he asked this, my heart fluttered. 'I'm just sitting on it, Nat. I've no intention of rushing into anything. I'm just stockpiling compost onsite and waiting for the right time to start working it.' 'Well, would you like a hand?'

A few months earlier I was in a very different situation. I'd just handed over management of quite a large organic fruit and veg operation in the Adelaide Hills that I'd been running for the previous three years. The site had been overrun with weeds due to previous poor management and, with my eyes full of stars but a lack of experience, I'd attempted to steer it towards production. After sinking my life's savings into this project and spending three years trying to turn a profit, I'd eventually had to walk away from it, broke, despondent, with relationships strained and my health in tatters. I didn't want to repeat this experience, so I was in no rush to develop the little block of land in Mitchell Park that had been so generously offered to me.

Nat and I had met a few years earlier at a workshop run by the revered urban farmer, Michael Ableman. Michael was touring Australia, giving talks on his experiences running operations in California and Vancouver. Following Michael's talk, the organising group held an impromptu 'meeting in the park' for anyone interested in being involved in setting up an urban agriculture project in Adelaide. All the 'heads' I'd heard about were there: Nicole Brammy, Joel Catchlove, Nat Wiseman, Chris Day, representatives from Grow West – people already making headway into changing the local food system in SA. I was just a hack who'd learned to grow my own corn for the love of the freshness and sweet, sweet flavour. When I told Nat about my farm in the hills after the meeting, he asked me if I enjoyed it. I told him that I did but I'd much rather grow food closer to where it was being eaten. This is when Nat asked me to come along to the Friends of the Earth 'city farm' project being spearheaded by himself and Graham Brookman from the Food Forest. This project was eventually quashed by the Adelaide City Council, citing soil contamination and resistance to proposals for a fence to be installed around the farm within the Parklands. Fortunately, Nat and I stayed in contact after this and became quite good friends.

It was a few years later when, as my large project south of Adelaide was winding down, one of the Adelaide growing gurus, Diana Bickford, asked me to meet with her and a few of the other young growers, to talk about forming a network to support all the new growers popping up around the traps.

Di has hands perfectly suited to digging in soil. With tough skin like a farmer, short fingers and incredibly gentle movements, she handles the largest, highest-quality and most-diverse range of certified organic seedlings I've ever come across. Naturally, she meets scores of people at her market stalls both in the Adelaide Showgrounds and up in the Hills at Stirling, and her farm is a magnet for aspiring growers to volunteer at and to get their own hands dirty. Di is a linchpin of the whole Adelaide growers' community. I met Di at the insistence of a friend's mother (a keen veggie gardener) and when I introduced myself, Di responded with, 'I've heard about you. There's a few other growers around the traps that I'd like to get together, a bit like the program [of peer support for regenerative farmers] that Allsun farm has running.

It's called 'Growing the Growers'. Here's the website, have a look and tell me what you think.'

Anyone even remotely interested in growing their own food in the city has a map of vacant urban blocks in their mind. Good aspect, no trees, alluvial soil, close to home – perfect for a little veg operation. The problem lies in finding the owner of the land and then striking a deal that suits both parties. This 'block at Mitchell Park' had come to my attention via another well-connected and community-minded matriarch, Beth Mylius. Beth and her late partner, Ray, had asked me to help them tidy up around their home. It was over a cup of tea and cake that Beth asked me, 'Apart from the farm in Meadows, what else are you interested in, Steven?' I explained about the Urban Farm group and Nat Wiseman's vision for an urban agriculture project in Adelaide, to which she replied, 'Now somebody sent me an email about offering some land up for a garden recently. Let me just go see if I can find it.' With that, she took her cuppa into her study only to emerge a few minutes later saying, 'I've just sent the lady a response asking if I can connect you two.'

The response came within a week. The landowners and I met on-site within a fortnight, a rental agreement was struck, whereby I keep the land free of weeds so the council has no reason to complain and I get to use the land for free! I contacted Nat immediately to tell him about the site, to which he responded, 'How big is it?' 'It's 230 square metres', I said. 'Hmm, it's a bit too small.' I remember thinking 'Well, in the state I'm in, it's too big for me to work alone!'

My plan was to slowly build up the resources I needed on-site, sheet mulch with cardboard and try to get the wild oat weed problem under control that way. When I took control of the site in late autumn, it looked like a wheat field as the oats had been cut down to stubble by the landowners. Along the back fence was an ancient grapevine creeping into the plot. The only other weed on-site was blackberry nightshade and, as this had been a huge nuisance at my previous farm, I made it my duty to carefully pull every single one out, tiny little fruits intact. There were also three tree stumps on site: one large one on the eastern boundary and two smaller ones in the middle.

I knew it would be advantageous to get some history on the site. I trawled through the council's land-use history and asked the elderly

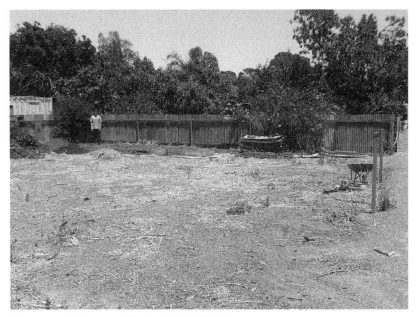

Figure 10.1. The vacant block at Mitchell Park. Photo courtesy of Steven Hoepfner.

neighbours as they walked past if they could remember what had happened there. One bloke in particular, a Mitchell Park native in his eighties, told me that it had been a 'bush block' since he could remember, it hadn't even had a shed on it. And the large stump belonged to a giant lemon-scented gum. Research in the council's archives showed that it was only in the 1950s that housing was rolled out through the area, with the Housing Trust taking the majority of the blocks. Prior to that, the area was market gardens. It was once referred to as 'the garden of Adelaide'. I couldn't believe it! Because of the nearby Sturt River, the soil underneath the site was alluvial floodplain.

Up until 1838, the land was sparsely settled and the river flowed without interruption, supporting life and land as it had done for thousands of years. The river has a name from way back then: 'Warripari', meaning 'windy place by the river'. It was an important area for the Kaurna people, being full of resources, having a mild climate and with the river being a regular site for travel, camping and foraging.

It was early 2012 when Nat, Kate Washington, her partner Genki and I finally found time for a tour of my recently finished project in the hills and then a visit to Di's farm to flesh out the details of this 'growers' network' we'd been talking about. It had also been a while since I had seen Nat so we had a bit to catch up on. His project to get a city farm established in the Adelaide Parklands had been quashed and he was obviously still coming to terms with that, so when he asked me about the Mitchell Park site, I was surprised. 'I thought you said it was too small?' I asked him. 'Well, it's bigger than my home garden and I just want to start practicing what I've learned...' (I can't really remember what he said after this, I was so incredibly excited to have the opportunity to work alongside Nat Wiseman!) We made plans to catch up again and work through the details. Nat asked if there was anyone else keen to be involved. There was.

One night a few weeks earlier, my good friend Brett had dropped in to my house unexpectedly, having just come from a sustainable houses meeting in the city. He kept asking me about the block at Mitchell Park and when I was going to start working it. I'll never forget how Brett, always bright and positive, was moping and despondent that night. I asked him how the meeting had gone and he replied, 'Everyone just kept arguing about the best building techniques, but no one spoke about doing anything with them. They can't see how urgent this all is. I had to leave because it was bringing me down. I don't know, man, all I want to do now is grow food!'

Brett, Nat and I met a few weeks later at Nat and his partner Jess' home in Goodwood. We agreed that, at this small scale, the farm would barely make enough to pay for itself, let alone a wage. As this could only be considered a hobby, we called it a hobby farm, decided how we would split the costs and returns (costs equally, returns as per hours accrued), then we made a map of the site, worked out the best bed layout, set a date in the diary and began removing tree stumps and planning to build a fence along the street frontage. A cyclone mesh fence was decided on – that way pedestrians could see in but knew that they couldn't just walk in (we saw plenty of well-meaning people accidentally trample beds during the years that followed). By the time we were ready for the compost delivery, the autumn rains had started and the site was awash with wild oat seedlings. It was perfect really, the grass seedlings were acting like a green manure and we were getting rid of the main weed problems in one fell swoop. As the soil hadn't been turned over for at least fifty years, we figured there wouldn't be any other weed problems. And, we were right! One other thing we did at Nat's insistence was to get a soil sample taken to see what its makeup was. The results showed that the soil was lacking in nitrogen and boron, but everything else was within the range suggested for veggie production! We knew we were standing on a rare bit of ground.

The next thing to do was to increase the organic soil matter, so we calculated that the site would require about 10 tonnes of compost to be rotary tilled through to get it 'alive' again. We put an order in with a local compost wizard and asked that the delivery be made the following week. Since we were trying to get the site ready for an autumn planting, we had also begun putting up our fence. We'd procured enough second-hand cyclone mesh to run across the street frontage, so Brett knocked up some gates and posts and we began installing everything. It was only late in the day when the truck of compost arrived that we realised we'd made it very difficult to drive a

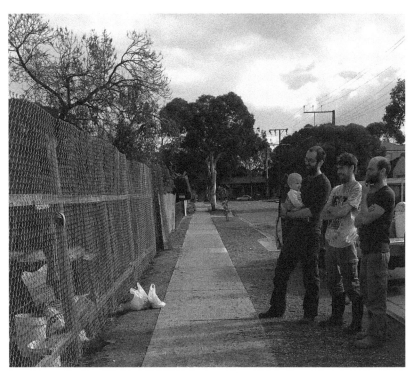

Figure 10.2. Nat (holding son Oliver), Steve and Brett admiring the new fence at the Wagtail Farm site. Photo courtesy of Jess Sanguesa.

10-tonne tip truck onto the site! Luckily, the compost wizard had also trained at the Kenworth school of ballet and was able to 'tiptoe' his rig through the gates on a 45-degree angle and dump the precious humus-enriching black gold close to the centre of the patch. This meant far less wheelbarrow work and spreading for us.

While the compost was being tilled into the soil, I remarked to Nat, 'Hey, there's that old willie wagtail that we always see here'. Nat looked up from his rake and without missing a beat, casually remarked, 'Perhaps that's what we should call the place: Wagtail Urban Farm'. The willie wagtail *(Rhipidura leucophrys)* is known in the local Kaurna tongue as *tjin tjin*, which means 'the gossip' or 'the messenger'. I like to think that our little farm heralds a message to the people that pass it by on foot or in their cars. Where did your food come from and how will it get there when we run out of fossil fuels?

Compost and fertiliser mixed in, beds shaped and levelled, we were ready to start planting the seedlings we'd been growing at Nat and Jess' place. At this stage, we didn't have any customers, a market, a retail outlet or any other method to move the produce that would be coming from the hundreds of seedlings we were about to plant! Nor did we have irrigation on-site as the mains water hadn't been connected yet! What we did have was a list of friends and family interested in the produce and a local fortnightly co-op that we could sell our wares at: enough potential mouths to eat perhaps a tenth of what we were likely to produce if we had a bad crop. By the looks of it, we weren't about to lose a single plant.

Surprisingly, every time we planted seedlings, it would either be raining as we planted or it would rain that night. This happened over a series of weeks, negating any need for water on-site until finally the mains were connected. There seemed to be a string of fortuitous happenings bringing Wagtail Urban Farm into fruition.

One such occasion was about a month after our first plantings, when we decided to have our first open day to coincide with Fair Food Week, 2013. We sent the word out through our networks and planned a whole Saturday of activities, demonstrations and tours. The day was a huge success with many hands making the events flow seamlessly. I'll never forget the feeling of having someone ask for a lettuce, spinach, tatsoi or other leafy green and being able to dart over

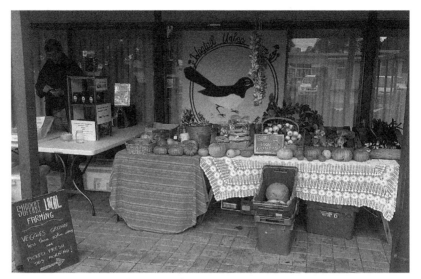

Figure 10.3. The Wagtail Farm market stall. Photo courtesy of Steven Hoepfner.

beds to harvest it for them on the spot. It really felt like the way things should be! During the day, I was approached by a woman named Aasha, who explained to Nat and me that she'd set up a community market in Glenelg that offered a fresh food co-op, with a membership of about 120 people. She said that Wagtail would be 'a perfect fit'. We had so much produce that we could easily service two markets a week. We set out a rotating market roster and began our new lives as urban farmers.

We continued like this for about a year, with Nat documenting inputs, produce, planting schedules and plant maturity rates. Finally, he decided that he was ready to start operating at a much larger scale. At the same time, he was presented with an offer that he couldn't refuse, a few acres inside an animal-proof fence on an eco-village south of Adelaide – with unlimited water! This was the beginnings of The Village Greens of Willunga Creek (commonly known as 'Village Greens'). Nat and the crew at Village Greens are really leading the way in regenerative agriculture here in South Australia.

It was around this time that Brett also decided that urban farming wasn't for him. Brett left Wagtail to focus on his newly forming family and a role working on the grounds at a school, but his legacy lives on at Wagtail, especially as he wrote the farm name over the gates.

Continuing on at Wagtail wasn't a hard decision but it hasn't been without its trials. Lonely, frosty morning harvests, people dumping their green waste onsite, irrigation and crop failures, floods, vermin and weird seasonal variations keep me on my toes, but it's all been worthwhile for the community and individual benefits (see figure 10.4, colour insert). Local councils now use the site for tours and visits; school groups come to see how growing food in the suburbs can work; community groups interested in sustainable living come to be inspired; volunteers come along and learn valuable tips on upping their home production; Permaculture Design Certificate students have visited to see a model of urban agriculture in the suburbs; soil scientists are using the site to measure the value of organic inputs on soil health; and our fortnightly market stall at the Organic Corner Store in Glenelg keeps feeding people with ethically grown and nutrient dense produce that has travelled fewer than 7 kilometres. Plus, I get access to the pick of the crop, so the love I pour into the soil nourishes me too. It's a no-brainer really!

But one of the most amazing benefits that Wagtail offers is the healing quality of getting back to the soil. A retired farmer once

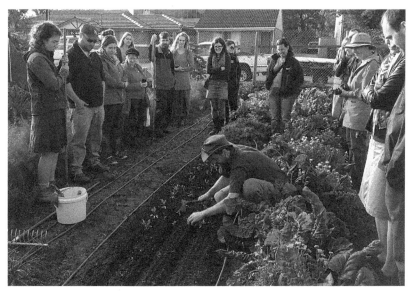

Figure 10.5. Steve demonstrating planting at Wagtail Farm for a Permaculture Design Certificate group from the Food Forest. Photo courtesy of Brett Young.

stopped at the gate on his walk along the street, as he often did, to chat. He noticed our pinpoint seeder leaning against the fence and became mesmerised, his eyes glassed over as he picked it up and then recounted how he used to tow a much larger version along behind his tractor when he worked the land back in his youth. His reverie was palpable and that moment wasn't lost on me. He quite obviously valued those days of growing food.

Wagtail offers many stories like this one, folk of all kinds connecting with the earth: a Kenyan woman drooling over our ripe cape gooseberries over the fence; a family from the Middle East teaching us you can eat the leaves of the Rosella plant *(Hibiscus sabdariffa)* and collecting bucket loads of them for use at home (we just grew them for the flowers!); our Chinese neighbours trading their pumpkins for our Daikon radish; and even an ex-convict reminiscing about his days in the prison garden!

Maybe the most touching connection so far has been the young lad who came to Adelaide after suffering a family tragedy while travelling overseas. Having worked in high-end kitchens in Asia all his life, he was amazed to stumble upon Wagtail while visiting friends in Mitchell Park. After making some enquiries, he got in touch and asked to come along and volunteer. Watching this young man taste, smell and touch the produce fresh from the earth was humbling to me. His surgical discernment of the flavours on offer reminded me of how little I sense and know about these plants, while he has been getting to know what the parent plants of the produce he's been using all these years look like. Being together in the garden was incredibly educational for both of us and it reminds me that the value of growing food isn't restricted to just physical nourishment.

Wagtail is still evolving and growing
Plans for Wagtail's future include installing a permanent toilet on-site and a small roofed structure over the veg prep area so that we can convert it to a 'classroom' for workshops for people wanting to take their productivity to the next level. There's also plans to make Wagtail's secret ingredient, its complete organic fertiliser, available to the rest of the world. But slowly, slowly! Rampant growth is rarely healthy and tends not to last for long…

Chapter 11

Melbourne City Rooftop Honey

Vanessa Kwiatkowski and Mat Lumalasi

The words 'urban agriculture' instantly bring to mind images of the textbook hipster or the army of inner-urban warriors competing to squeeze more mouse melons and heirloom tomatoes onto their 600-square-metre vacant parcel of land, courtyard or balcony. As much as it may be an amusing image, it does have a positive serious side.

Consumers today are really reconnecting with their food and food-supply chain. Fewer than four generations ago, our ancestors lived through the Great Depression, in many cases desperately clinging to any viable food source. This was a time when being careless with food and resources simply wasn't an option. Nothing was wasted and, for many, 'nose to tail' eating was a survival strategy. These days, we frequently see 'nose to tail' on the menu of venues trying to show more respect for food by not wasting a morsel.

As time went on and the global economy recovered, we went through a period of great economic and industrial development, leading to the 'era of convenience' when supermarkets arrived. We didn't have to worry about preserving and eating in season, we got what we wanted when we wanted it and it was all laid out in front of us in perfect plastic-wrapped portions. Along the journey of modernisation, we lost touch with our connection to the food we eat and, some might say, we lost touch with ourselves.

Now, we see a certain irony in the world, where countries like Cuba, living under embargo and excluded from international trade, are forced to be self-sufficient and bring food production all the way into the heart of their cities. Western consumerism is expanding all around them and they are left dreaming of the day when they can be a part of that picture, while our own urban-agriculture movement is wanting the opposite. More Australians are resisting a duopoly of supermarkets dictating what farmers get paid and that are selling genetically modified and pesticide-laden produce as well as highly processed 'foods'. This reminds us of the saying, 'if your grandmother wouldn't recognise it, you shouldn't be eating it'. The Cuban and Australian food systems have evolved over time in very different ways and both point to opportunities as well as challenges.

For our part, we saw a need to revive a craft that was somewhat dying in ageist hands. We felt it was imperative to reconnect people with the food-supply chain by linking our resilient, sustainable city and suburbs with urban beekeeping.

When we started the project in 2010, we saw it as an opportunity to raise awareness of the various threats faced by the honeybee and to be part of the greater worldwide effort to help. It started as a basic idea that was intended to be a weekend hobby project, though it quickly gained so much more momentum than we could ever have imagined. With some lucky timing, we found ourselves on the crest of a wave and Melbourne City Rooftop Honey was born.

Even though our project is inherently local, our message has a much broader reach. What we do not only seeks to address issues of sustainability, it also aims to raise awareness of the importance of bees and the various threats they face globally.

By placing hives on the roof spaces of businesses, cafés, restaurants, hotels and individual gardens in and around Melbourne, we have reduced the distance between production and plate from kilometres to mere metres (see figures 11.1a and 11.1b, colour insert). In doing so, our work is intended to inspire others to think about the broader environmental implications of their actions and choices.

We see our harvest of honey as a great symbol for high-quality local produce, but Melbourne City Rooftop Honey also operates as a social enterprise that aims to help grow communities as well as demonstrate social and environmental responsibility and ethical food production.

Our work also demonstrates that we are part of an elaborate ecosystem that depends on bees more than they depend on us. While crops vary in how much they rely on or respond to pollination by bees, in Australia, around 65 per cent of agricultural production depends on pollination by European honeybees. There are thirty-five industries that depend on honeybee pollination for most of their production, with some crops, such as almonds, apples, pears and cherries, almost entirely dependent. These crops ultimately comprise a very large proportion of the food that we all eat: around one in three mouthfuls![1]

Due to the large number of wild European honeybees in Australia, the vital role that pollination plays is not widely recognised or valued, and only a small proportion of agricultural producers manage the process themselves. Mostly, this is done through paid pollination, in which a fruit or nut producer pays a beekeeper to put beehives among the trees.

There are several threats to bee populations globally, especially the emergence in 2006–07 of Colony Collapse Disorder, which saw widespread decline and even loss of entire honeybee colonies in the USA and Europe. Exotic pests such as the Varroa mite, which is yet to become established in Australia, potentially pose a very serious threat to our honeybees and their pollination services. In light of these challenges, it's essential to recognise the critical role that honeybees play in the sustainability of the food-supply system.

The rooftop honey idea itself was one of those 'moments of clarity' emerging out of practical local experience and information gleaned from other sources. Vanessa had been reading articles online and in our local *Diggers Club* magazine, as well as books like *The Urban Food Revolution* and *City Farmer: Adventures in Urban Food Growing*, and had become concerned about food, food production and people's loss of connection to it as well as the worldwide decline in bees.[2] At the same time, as a keen gardener, she was already growing a lot of our own food (we have a big raised veg patch and greenhouse on yes… a 600-square-metre block). We already had our own bees in our suburban backyard and one morning Vanessa woke up and said, 'let's take the bees to the city'.

The connection between the restaurants and placing hives on roofs emerged from reading online about how chefs needed to make more sustainable choices for the future. We had read studies about bees in the city being healthier and about urban beekeeping thriving in places like Paris, London, Toronto, San Francisco and New York City.[3] Suddenly, it seemed logical to do something that was being practiced in many European countries – why not here? It was our opportunity to be proactive rather than reactive: 'prevention is better than cure'.

However, our concept is different to a lot of other urban beekeeping movements. We not only share honey with our supporters, we also share knowledge, connect people and create a sense of community. We do this via workshops, public talks, school group educational tours of our hives and in-store 'meet the producer' events at retailers. We've done a host of radio interviews and TV appearances. We've also placed hives with various community groups in and around the city and the suburbs. The honey from these hives goes directly back to the people to consume or to raise funds for initiatives or charity. We

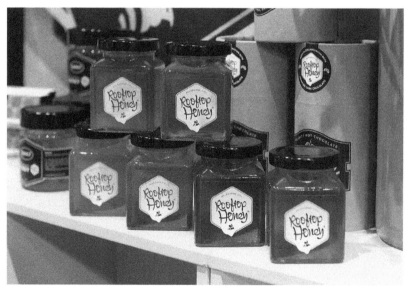

Figure 11.2. Rooftop Honey jars stocked by Clementine's, near a hive site on Degraves Street in Melbourne. Photo courtesy of Anneliese Henjak.

show our appreciation to community-funded programs by supporting other small businesses and collaborating on projects. We also donate to independent enterprises such as Cinema Nova and local radio stations 3RRR FM and 3MBS for fundraising events like Radiothons.

The local community also benefits by gaining access to some true 'local' produce – a great tasting honey, which is raw, unblended and unique to each site. Each jar has a terroir reflecting the flora that has been foraged in the local areas.

What started out as a small hobby project is now a full-time role for us both. Beekeeping is largely seasonal here in Victoria, with our season being spring until autumn. We are continually working on making what started out as a hobby into a sustainable business that keeps the roof over our head. At the same time, we stay true to our original ethical motivations behind the enterprise. This is sometimes tricky to balance, but our efforts are often reinforced by way of the overwhelming support from the people of Melbourne – individuals who offer their places for hive adoptions as well as businesses wanting to offer sponsorships.

We now have hundreds of businesses and individuals on a waiting list to get involved and it has been amazing to see the interest in bees and beekeeping in suburbia flourish. This is our barometer of impact. It is hard for us to count the flowers, but we are sure, if we did so, we would find that our 6.5 million bees must have made some difference in the greening of Melbourne. There is a whole chain of environmental impacts and the flow-on effects are huge. Birds and dragonflies are following the bees and coming back into our urban environment. Bees are sourcing nectar from their local environment and providing a priceless pollination service.

One area in which we have seen evidence of a shift in public perception is swarm season. Bees were traditionally seen as pests by the public when they swarmed and local councils would often opt for the fast and easy solution of extermination. It is only in recent years that people have realised their importance, so rather than destroy the 'pests', we are now being called to collect these swarms or colonies and give them a more suitable home. We first check their temperament by placing them in a holding apiary and, if they are friendly enough, they go back into the community to be managed. If they are unfriendly, we look to 're-queen' them.

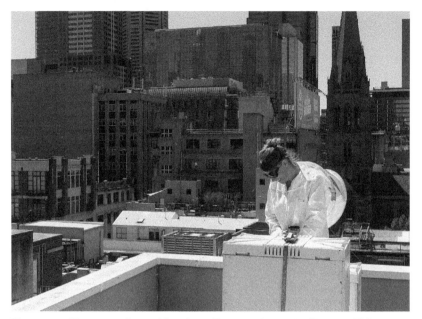

Figure 11.3. Vanessa tends to a hive above Degraves Street, Melbourne CBD. Photo courtesy of Anneliese Henjak.

Throughout history, bees have been one of our environmental indicators, but over time, urban people have become somewhat disconnected from nature and bees. Some people don't realise how important they truly are. Personally, we think it is necessary to link the bees to the sustainable existence of humans as a spur to action. We don't have a choice on this issue and, unfortunately, often we don't do anything about issues until the situation is bordering on crisis.

We see honey as a by-product of keeping happy, healthy bees. Bees are so industrious and they work so hard and we believe it is unethical to take all the honey from them and feed them sugar syrup like some commercial and hobby practices do (and are even taught to do). We only take the excess when the nectar flow is on and always leave them with enough of their own food stores to ensure their future survival.

Humans have a basic right to access fresh food. It shouldn't be just for the privileged or wealthy and individual companies should never own the rights to a seed or plant. People who provide food for themselves should be encouraged, as it takes a great burden off many expensive systems like health, transport and global warming.

We encourage you to do anything you can to be more environmentally mindful and to connect with your local community. Humans are social creatures too: we need one another; we need support, encouragement and to know we are not alone in the fight to help our sick planet. These efforts will keep you inspired and the flow-on effect will eventually lead people from a consumerist mindset to a harmonious global world and ecosystem.

We don't see ourselves as being a major player or hugely influential. We are just two people doing what we can, trying to make a change one rooftop at a time. It's the bees who deserve the credit.

Chapter 12

Farming is Punk!

Joel Orchard

Farming is punk. It is grounded in defiance and rooted in community.

My first taste of food systems activism was in 2011 through a Greenpeace campaign against the genetically modified canola feed being imported predominantly for battery farms and the broiler chicken supply chain for the fast-food industry. An entertaining foray into non-violent direct action had me cuffed and stuffed in the back of a paddy wagon wearing a giant chicken suit. The irony of the caged chicken was not lost. Apparently, during the 'performance' inside the Australasian Poultry Convention on the Gold Coast where we had wildly paraded and chanted, I had inadvertently flapped a wing and knocked off a police officer's hat.

A minor misdemeanour but it was one that set the wheels in motion for me and opened my mind to the potent connection between environmental activism, politics and food. So many of the simple realities of my childhood have become far more relevant with my new lens of understanding. The food system has been broken for a long time.

I grew up in south west Victoria, one of the richest dairy farming regions in Australia, but it certainly wasn't the farmers getting rich. Stories of farmers pouring their milk down the drain were common even twenty years ago. 'Home brand' milk was in, Nestlé had just converted the local processing facility to produce powdered milk for the export market to the rising middle class in China, the local Dairy Cooperative was struggling to maintain viability and the Big Dairy corporates were shuffling their shares in a grab for the global dairy market… meanwhile farmers were being gouged on the price of milk.

Our conventional country-town block was surrounded by farms and paddocks. We had a good selection of fruit trees, a vegetable garden producing carrots that tasted like carrots; tomatoes that tasted like tomatoes; peach, nectarine and apple trees you could climb and enough corn to fill the freezer each season. We gleaned roadsides for blackberries, plums and quinces and we had a healthy larder of preserved fruits in neat rows of the ubiquitous glass jars: Fowlers Vacola with little labels. The surrounding farmland has since been replaced (as have so many peri-urban farms) with neat rows of house blocks as a result of urban sprawl.

I spent several years as a staunch, radical vegan, dumpster diving my way through university, and had a micro farm in pots outside my third-floor dorm room. Perhaps those were the signs that I was not to fit into the traditional food-consumer paradigm.

We grew an awesome vegetable plot in the front and backyards of a share house in inner-city Melbourne. A most impressive stand of sunflowers was a Richmond highlight for the best part of the season. I gifted cut flowers to brighten faces and traded blooms for home-grown daikon at the commission houses' community gardens in Little Saigon on Victoria Street.

At this time, I was working as a fruiterer for an organic produce store and café in the city and doing the twice-weekly run to the Melbourne wholesale markets to order and collect produce for the shop. Here, I got first-hand experience of the scale and complexities of the wholesale fresh-produce distribution system for Victoria. This market is of epic proportions. It's a space of wild activity accentuated by the ruckus of forklifts travelling at breakneck speeds, with trucks and pallets packed high with fresh produce from around the country.

I got to talk to farmers, distributors, merchants, marketeers and the many hands of this dynamic and complicated food chain.

In 2008, Melbourne had all but run out of water due to the drought and we DIY-diverted grey water to our veggie garden. That year there was enough media attention on the increase in cases of gastro to cast doubt on this practice and we let the gardening go for the season.

In 2009, I left the city with my science degree and moved to Bendigo. That year the drought had become so bad that Lake Wendouree dried out and caught on fire. This was no place to grow food.

Growing food as a primary function of living a sustainable lifestyle had now become such a high priority for me that a more drastic move was required, and not long after I landed in the Northern Rivers wet subtropics. The annual 2000 millimetres of rain outdoes most places in Australia's rainfall totals and learning to grow food and subsistence farm in this environment had its own challenges.

I took a job at Santos Organics, whose long legacy of involvement in the organics retail industry stretched back to the Aquarian festival and migration of hippies to the region in the 1970s. As the ethics and procurement officer, I delved further into my understanding of food and policies, issues of localisation, preservatives, additives and packaging.

We used this platform to educate consumers and campaign on issues such as child trafficking in the chocolate industry, rainforest destruction for palm oil and the boycott of Japanese products in support of *Sea Shepherd*. Food was a powerful tool for consumer democracy.

What had started off for simple satisfaction and as a simple veggie patch at home had turned into an obsession of sorts. I revelled in this new climate where it seems you could grow just about everything all year-round – and that's exactly what I did.

I also applied my interest in science and research and pored through books and literature while trying to understand the community's well-developed alternative food system. With an extensive network of farmers markets and a community with a high level of food literacy, it seemed that an engaged and informed consumer base was making enough choices about its food that the market for organic cafes, organic farmers markets and organic retail stores producing cleaning products, clothes, cosmetics and family products had developed to meet to the growing demand.

This region was the birthplace of the organics, permaculture and seed savers movements in Australia. Its long association with the virtues of permaculture and a self-sufficient lifestyle hovered at a friendly distance for the conventional farming community, yet it still benefited from the services and infrastructure associated with the region's rich farming history.

Tree changers had moved to the area and adopted revegetation and bush regeneration programs. Small-scale farming and organic agriculture erupted alongside the declining traditional agricultural industries. It was within this dichotomy that I recognised the opportunity that ecological farming offered as a mechanism to preserve and protect the region's biodiversity. With the region's rich history of environmentalism, an established 'clean and green' culture and the locals' appreciation for the area's lush ecological richness, it seemed to me that we needed an industry to support and consolidate the local conservation movement.

I also recognised that being on the fringe of Australia's fastest growing urban corridor (the Gold Coast and Brisbane) offered major advantages and opportunities from a farming perspective. Rich volcanic soils, plentiful rainfall and the potential for huge crop diversity meant that the region represented an enormous opportunity to act as a significant food bowl for these rapidly growing urban populations.

To me, the development of an ecological agriculture industry had the potential to bring together the greenie sentiments that had defined the region, utilise a gross waste of amazing fertile farmland and contribute to tackling youth unemployment. So, for a region with amazing natural resources, existing infrastructure and a significant consumer base, it was confronting to find that there simply wasn't a thriving and growing agricultural industry.

What I found just under the surface was the glaring issue of an ageing farmer population. I soon realised that this was not only a local and national issue, it was worldwide.

Future Feeders

I set to the task of exploring this issue of an ageing farmer population and the socioeconomic conundrum that had left the small-scale farming industry in the region insular and stagnant, with few opportunities for employment, fewer opportunities for skills development and mentorship, and next to no new or young farmers to talk with.

The industry had become quite dependent on WWOOFers (Willing Workers on Organic Farms) as a readily available supply of free labour, which went hand-in-hand with the local backpacker community.

There were multiple barriers in the way of would-be young farmers. Land prices had spiked out of control, so affordable farmland was non-existent for start-up farmers. The farmers markets had locked themselves down into a model that restricted trading and opportunities to new entrants. The much larger issue of the family farming model, which had seen the traditional succession plan of passing farms from parents to kids, had failed. Young people moved out of the region in search of jobs and opportunities in the cities and the farmland was quickly being bought up for rural lifestyle, holiday homes and speculative investment.

I had started a small market garden, taking over the neighbouring paddock and teaming up with the landowner of the property where I lived, who was already near to retirement and trying his hand at garlic. We soon moved into ginger and turmeric as less labour-intensive cash crops.

In developing a biological farm management plan, I found my calling when reading Fukuoka's *One Straw Revolution*.[1] On these pages, I read that farming was more than a practice – it was a philosophy for healthy living and a reminder that, clearly, our future depends on reconnecting with the natural world, knowing our food, regenerating our land and strengthening our communities. Many more books, films and stories followed to cement the ideas, principles and belief that farming truly holds the key to many of society's economic and ecological injustices, from deforestation and soil degradation, to rebuilding ecosystems and replenishing soil carbon.

Wendel Berry's foreword to the book said it all: 'We cannot isolate one aspect of life from another. When we change the way we grow our food, we change our food, we change society, we change our values.' It was a drive for change that propelled me into farming.

I found myself enamoured by the poetry of reverence for nature that also described a meticulous and scientific approach to the fundamental connection and dependence that we each have to nature though our food: a connection that was quite clearly being lost through our urbanisation and convenience culture. But, while Fukuoka advocated a 'do-nothing' natural farming system, I pictured a 'do-something' farming system.

For me, the problems with the food system meant that not only had the *culture* been taken out of *agriculture* since the green revolution, but also that mass production, distribution and commodification of the food system had taken most of the nourishment from what we eat and left us with plastic-wrapped, manufactured, food-like products. In turn, the perpetuation of the system required immense land destruction, fossil fuel and energy use, soil degradation and chemical application.

Farming thus became a vehicle of change for me, one that enabled me to combine a passion for social activism and environmentalism, and gave me a chance to connect with the earth and restore a story of health through food.

In every way, it seemed to me that we needed to bring together eaters and farmers to ensure that deep and tangible connection with the earth. The more we could bring food to the forefront of people's minds, the more they would see the impact of the traditional agriculture system around them on the landscape and demand not only an alternative for their bodies, but for the planet.

We don't need more mass-produced, large-scale, broad-acre, monoculture, genetically modified, globalised-farming production. We need a future of networked, small-scale, localised, agro-ecologies nourishing the soil, giving back to the land and feeding our communities. This is what Future Feeders represents. Yet, what I saw was a stereotyped vision of the farmer that is deeply embedded in the Australian psyche and is far less inspiring: it's a male figure who is solemn, weathered and alone.

I wanted to shift gears and punk the farming model out with a DIY attitude, blend in collaboration for resource and skills sharing, and explore appropriate technology and cooperation. I wanted to embrace the far-broader skill set of the digital native generation, with media and communication and networking.

I wanted to engage young farmers in the possibility of sustainable land management through innovation and self-empowerment. I wanted to build a platform that worked like an ecology, diverse and self-supporting, that captured the change-makers' spirit, to propel young people into meaningful careers in the local food economy.

It was happening elsewhere – and I have taken huge inspiration from initiatives in the USA, such as the Greenhorns, the National Young Farmers Coalition, the Farmers Guild, Kiss the Soil and many other awesome platforms.

There are so many barriers for first-generation farmers, who are now coming from urban backgrounds and who haven't inherited the family farm with systems and infrastructure and equipment in place. In my mind, we are already ten years too late – the average farmer is nearly sixty and the policymakers haven't seemed to notice that farmers under the age of forty are in decline. We need a grass-roots solution to getting young folks onto the land and getting skills growing food through viable dynamic business models.

We rallied the first group of Future Feeders in early 2014 to tackle an abandoned banana farm just outside town and we made plans to take a lease on a 1.5-acre block of land at the Mullumbimby Community Gardens to run as a market garden.

None of us had worked on a banana farm before. It was punishing work and a naive dive head first into a project that held little hope for decent financial return – yet it was a starting point that filled our need and enthusiasm to have some action in the field. It gave us an opportunity to come together and share ideas and, while we felt like we might have been saving this one farm, it was just one of many in the region that had been let decay for one reason or another.

When we started to share our story and get some media attention, there was a flood of offers – abandoned mango farms, lemon myrtle plantations, coffee plantations, market gardens and acres and acres and acres of disused, surplus farmland all around the Northern Rivers. The prospects were all a little overwhelming! We re-grouped and staked out a market garden at the community gardens for ourselves and began the process of a low-cost, low-risk experiential farm from which to grow food, our skills and the Future Feeders movement (see figure 12.1, colour insert).

From this point, the experiments began: experiments with crops and the development of an identity. Farming really was only one part of the journey as was marketing, distribution and building awareness

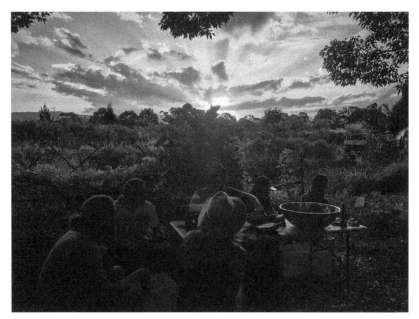

Figure 12.2. Young Farmers Network gathering at Future Feeders. Photo courtesy of Joel Orchard.

and a community. We began our associations with the broader food movement and, feeling somewhat ostracised from the local farming community, we reached out to the small-scale producers and family-farming networks such as Food Connect, the Family Farmers United Network and Australian Food Sovereignty Alliance.

The original core team dispersed over time into other operations and we also began to find a common connection with other young farmers throughout the region. The Northern Rivers Young Farmers Alliance formed as a result and offered a communications platform and an extended peer-support network for the new and young farmers of the region. We began a series of field days and we use a social media group for capacity building, information sharing, opportunities and networking.

In evolution

Over the last two years, the market garden has evolved into a Community Supported Agriculture (CSA) subscription model and has developed and trialled a local Participatory Guarantee System (PGS) (see figure 12.3a and 12.3b, colour insert). Seeing the farm as an opportunity to fulfil the need for platforms and pathways into the local farming industry, I am now partitioning the farm into smaller and more manageable units to offer as a 'micro farm incubator' within a twelve-month internship program.

Building the farmer incubator model has been the goal from the outset and it feels like progress to be able to move the farm on to fresh start-ups. It also provides me with some more freedom to begin tackling some of the more systemic issues and advocacy – I will now go back to my dream for the Future Feeders movement with a broader view to build a national support framework for our emerging young farmers.

What do I love most about farming?
Connecting people to food and the earth
Few things compare to having families turn up at the farm to collect their weekly produce with kids running full steam at the trellis of snow peas and cherry tomatoes.

Developing a relationship with nature
Sharing a space with an ecology and being involved in its daily ebbs and flows, and getting to know individual birds and frogs and snakes is an incredible experience.

I now have three to four generations of fairy wrens that have nested on the farm. They dance in the ute window and will sit on my boots when I rest in the shade. I know that when the red-breasted wrens pass through, it's the change of season to spring and that when the restless flycatchers turn up that autumn is on its way. I've met more species of native bees than I knew existed and made a connection with an incredible array of frogs.

Best of all, I have witnessed the development of a healthy, thriving ecology through the result of my labour. To turn a uniform weedy paddock into a habitat of such biodiversity has given me so much joy that the carrots, corn, tomatoes and broccoli seem secondary in importance. I'm confident that this is the way to grow food and to eat.

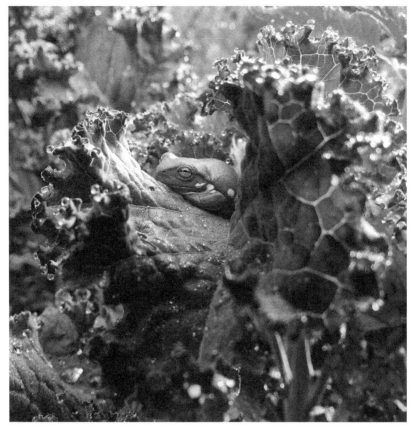

Figure 12.4. Friends on the farm: a green tree frog nestled in a curly kale leaf.
Photo courtesy of Joel Orchard.

Farming feels like something real
You really use your body as if that is how it was intended to be used. It's also a creative use of the mind through constant problem solving, designing and planning. I have never slept so well in all my life and I have hardly been sick. I know if I were better at business, my account would be richer, but the experience has certainly been rich!

Farming is punk
Farming is direct action and a reclaiming of something tangible. It also gives you complete control over what you eat, how it was produced and the impact of its production.

Call to action

So, from here, I am inviting young farmers to take action: to take inspiration and come together to resource and develop a platform to recognise and support Australia's young farmers.

Let us start a Future Feeders movement and vibrant young farmers network for our local food economies. Let us create an institution that represents a change in the farming culture with a groundswell of activity that generates a new narrative, grows jobs and opportunities, revitalises our rural communities and challenges economic models and limitations to ensure that the future is filled with fresh, organic vegetables, smiles and good health.

Chapter 13

Urban Food Street

Caroline Kemp

'We shape our houses, and afterwards, our buildings shape us.'
Winston Churchill

Suburban streets are the arteries of public life, the life blood of our daily existence and are linked intrinsically with our physical and social conceptions of 'home' and 'neighbourhood'. But what do they offer apart from a passage of movement from one life event to another? What should a neighbourhood be like aesthetically? What does it offer socially? How should it perform environmentally and who is ultimately responsible for shaping the vitality of its public life?

Contemporary, top-down models deliver culturally accepted, monolithic ideas of designed suburban space, aesthetically, functionally and economically. Residents occupy suburban space predictably, to the point that they live in and demand the banality of their urban surrounds in a perfect, one-size-fits-all type of way – effectively, a hegemonic mono-functionality.

My partner, Duncan, and I live in a mono-functional suburb in a sub-tropical regional town in Queensland. Our suburb is marked by wide swathes of turfed nature strip[1] zones, not uncommon in cities across Australia, where housing-estate land is carved up to ensure maximum sales gain, rather than positive liveability. We endured the unintended consequences of planned urban growth and the side effects, such as social suburban isolation. Then in 2009, spurred on by the high price of a single lime, we had a very simple idea. By planting a lime tree on the verge adjacent to our house, and inviting others to pick from future crops, we believed we could generate a life and vitality within our suburban street that was uncommon in the Australian suburban context. This gesture also offered a simple and effective solution to the issue of food miles and waste.[2]

It was an idea that was cemented for both of us during a trip to New York the following year, when we discussed the notion of 'neighbourhood' with a shop assistant on Bleecker Street, in Greenwich Village. Simple observations can be profound. Somehow in the sea of urban density that is New York, the people of Greenwich Village have managed to form an identity and connection around an understanding of 'neighbourhood' that is predominantly spatial in nature. These ideas of 'social collectivity', framed through dialogue about the urban form, were repeated to us on numerous occasions as we traversed the neighbourhoods of Manhattan Island; each time encompassing the same spatial qualities and understandings of the space in which people live. There are some fabulous makers of place and commentators on urban life who have called New York home, including Jane Jacobs and more recently the Project for Public Spaces (PPS),[3] as well as the office of urban designer Jan Gehl. Maybe what we were experiencing was linked to their collective presence across the city landscape. The discourse we encountered contained proud references to intimate neighbourhoods defined by a boundary, measured by walkable distances and animated by an eccentric street life. There is a sense of connection that comes from identifying with the 'neighbourhood'. In our experience, this is largely lacking in the Australian context. While Australian suburbia is unlike the densely populated urban form of Manhattan, it seemed feasible to us that the qualities of 'neighbourhood' were transferable to a suburban context.

Ideas of 'neighbourhood' and what a neighbourhood could offer, defined by spatial proximity rather than the more commonly used term 'community' (including the relationship between spatial quality and human occupation), started to form for both of us. Perhaps in a subconscious awareness of our dilemma, and following on from the 2009 idea to plant a lime tree, we had already planted the verge adjacent to our home with over a dozen citrus trees. If nothing else, we thought those trees might bring a social and environmental definition to the banal streets in which we lived.

Armed with a suite of civic engagement ideas from New York, we began referring to the citrus trees as *part* of an integrated suburban fabric. The citrus trees brought personality and a presence to our street and defined them as fundamentally different. Strategically identifying the planted precinct as 'neighbourhood' signalled our increased awareness of the impact that the urban form has on our collective quality of life. It also triggered ideas for some simple and inexpensive ways that bottom-up, people-focused and people-led design can enhance the quality of day-to-day existence.

The vast, turfed nature strips throughout our neighbourhood are part of a collective public amenity and an extension of our homes. They comprise a shared, dormant and under-utilised public space. However, through new interpretation of function, this space has the potential to host propositions that improve social connections, thereby offering tangible solutions at a local level to declining levels of physical and mental health. We had plenty of room within our suburban plot to plant the citrus trees, but this offered no solution to the health issues associated with suburban isolation, sedentary lifestyle or the environmental issues of food miles and waste.

The solution to this problem could be achieved while nurturing people with some of the freshest and most nutrient-dense food around. Urban Food Street™ is the outcome: an exercise in urban design and a direct challenge to the legacy thinking and outdated understandings that plague much of this country's contemporary suburban housing outcomes.[4]

Lessons learnt on a trip to South America in 2011 included observations of the historically low-income, informal settlement in Brazil, the *favela*. Freed from fixed and stereotypical ideas of how a place should look and function, the informal settlement reveals a number of design qualities, such as a walkable and lively street life and proximity to amenities that contribute to high levels of resilience in the face of daily adversity. Without romanticising the magnitude of problems associated with this type of settlement, urban designers such as Jan Gehl understand that characteristics such as 'proximity', 'scale', 'street life', 'flexibility' and 'personality' can contribute to a robust sense of place. Noting also that these attributes should be preserved in the face of future top-down civic intervention, it was these very design qualities that we saw value in replicating.[5] However, in order to achieve that in our suburban neighbourhood, we needed a catalyst.

Growing fresh fruit and vegetables on our verge demonstrates the potential of the informal and challenges an established view of suburbia and what suburbia as 'place' offers. It is an acknowledgement that the dominant presentation of suburban public space is highly prescribed in a way that denies the diversity that comes from progressive thinking. Our suburbia is also environmentally and socially unsustainable, making it inherently flawed for our contemporary and rapidly changing times.

We had no plans at the outset other than to allow the concept to evolve naturally and organically, to the extent that calling our first plantings 'a project' seems a little disingenuous. Our first plantings were just putting edible plant species into the ground in public spaces for the genuine enjoyment of all. They later became a design-thinking[6] response that spoke about the qualities of the 'informal' settlement, the *favela*, over the formality of the prescribed urban form to generate a new modality of thinking.

Bottom-up and free from traditional hierarchical structures and organisational procedures that are often associated with government initiatives and not-for-profit organisations, we were ten neighbourhood families that met once only, in 2009, to discuss the qualities associated with the type of neighbourhood in which we all wished to dwell. Human connection and cohesion topped the list of desirable qualities, with many also wanting our oldest neighbourhood residents to experience ageing-in-place[7].

We appropriated the concept of design ecology from Ken Maher's 2009 A. S. Hook address and used it to guide the direction of the project. Maher writes:

> *I believe designing in the future will need to be an organic process, an ecological process, where landscape and nature are integrated and interpreted. We need*

a new design ecology that reaches beyond economics and physics to embrace human senses and emotions, and to define an architecture that reflects life at a deeper level or, in Siegfried Gideon's words, 'the interpretation of a way of life valid for our period'. [8]

As a result of this way of thinking, we agreed the project would be de-structured and devoid of conventional organisational or structural expectation. The project was determined by a walkable boundary of eleven residential streets (cognisant of design for walkability) and about 220 households (approximately 1,000 people). We called it Food Street and continued on with daily living. We had no expectation the project would grow, morph or evolve into anything. We hoped it would demonstrate the capacity of design to subvert the forces that isolate people and privilege individual gain over collective benefit. We had no grand expectations.

By 2011, the verge citrus trees had grown substantially and were starting to produce good quantities of pesticide-free fruit. In order to chase the vibrant suburban street life we sought, Duncan and I resisted the urge to pick the lime crop that year. Instead, we promoted the idea, via handwritten messages on fence mounted chalkboards and casual conversations with neighbours, that if you lived in the neighbourhood, your next lime was only a short walk away. Anyone that lived within the eleven residential streets was invited to pick freely from that season's crop. Word got around the neighbourhood that the fruit was available to pick and slowly people started to catch on. It was such a fundamental shift from our status-quo suburban understanding of what a typical neighbourhood's physical and social dimension offered, that community participation required gentle encouragement.

Our fundamental aim for growing citrus (and later on a wide range of other food crops) on the street edge in the early days was therefore not about 'urban agriculture' at all, but rather about activating the street. We planted food-producing trees as a catalyst and then informally noted the changing ways in which people engaged with that space. We watched that space generate all sorts of interaction between all sorts of people. We referred to it as the 'social site' and, as the public space plantings spread across the precinct, we casually observed the differing factors of physicality that led to genuine forms of engagement between people throughout different streets. We transitioned to talking about the urban agriculture merits of the precinct some years on when we realised the abundance of good quality food that was being produced though the process of suburban activation.

Researchers have been writing for years about the correlation between contemporary Australian suburban housing developments and the rising rates of social isolation, poor mental and physical health and sedentary lifestyles. Australian architect Robin Boyd, in his seminal text *The Australian Ugliness*,[9] anticipated this in the 1960s. Although this was largely an attack on the aesthetics of Australian building design and planning, Boyd was a strong advocate of the significance of the connection between people and their dwelling/site. He also bemoaned the trend toward the wholesale copying of all things American, including vast tracts of cookie-cutter, profit-driven sub-divisions.

Economics aside (although economic issues are important and relevant), much of this can be broken down into an urban form issue. We desired an alternative to the contrived, lifeless outcomes that are delivered repeatedly across the Australian suburban landscape and applied mono-culturally through a prescription of top-down processes, regardless of individual place-based qualities. Activating our nature strip, informally but authentically, seemed the logical response.

We knew that if the project was to achieve and maintain activation, it had to do two things. Firstly, from a structural perspective, it had to yield bountiful quantities of fresh seasonal food grown by us and other neighbours, sufficient enough to be both rewarding and interesting and also public enough to be 'owned' as a collective resource by those in the neighbourhood. The project had to fundamentally relate to, and be a critical part of, their day-to-day existence; integrated as a suburban norm, informal and without the common socio-cultural expectations associated with participation or aesthetics.

Secondly, and most importantly (I can't emphasise this point enough), it had to be easy – that is, easy enough to engender interest, which ultimately leads to participation. Participation, ideally, is truly fluid, tailored according to lifecycle needs and specific abilities, enabling families to opt in and out as required. It is only through the application of design-thinking, taking ideas from the informal settlement and applying these across the site that we are able to see all aspects of the project as fluid.

Any individual or organisation can implement a project. That is the easy part. Usually projects fold once the hierarchical direction and/or funding is removed. Getting people to participate over the long term, while fostering project and membership growth, is the true challenge. This challenge is familiar to Dr Zoe Myers at the Urban Design Research Centre at the University of Western Australia, who notes that 'community cohesion is hard to implement or encourage from top-down initiatives, but highly sought after once established'.[10] Positive examples of projects that started at a community level and that are still highly active include the High Line in New York and CERES Community Environment Park in Melbourne.

People attract people. Delight is in the unexpected and the everyday. Maybe the noticeboard has been chalked with a new neighbourhood message. Maybe the verge-grown tropical stone fruit is almost ripe. Maybe the children from our local childcare centre are walking the streets and picking produce. All of these small and everyday acts nurtured local sensibilities, helping to create a place-based identity and providing reasons for people to connect with the physicality of their suburban surrounds, whilst gently encouraging active and healthy living.

Limes were now free when in season and other interesting things were happening around the streets of the Urban Food Street neighbourhood. Families from several streets away were walking the streets looking for produce, talking with one another when meeting on the street during an afternoon walk with the dog or their children; this was critically important. Those living around us were benefitting from the camaraderie that connection with others brings.

Importantly, by starting the process organically and evolving strategically through the application of design-thinking, the neighbourhood was producing incredibly high yields of free, non-sprayed, nature-strip-grown fresh fruit and vegetables (see figure 13.2, colour insert). As a nature-strip-based project that was funded without government or private sector money, it was doing what no local-government-led initiative or not-for-profit project had managed to do. And it was thriving. Replicated where appropriate (although it isn't

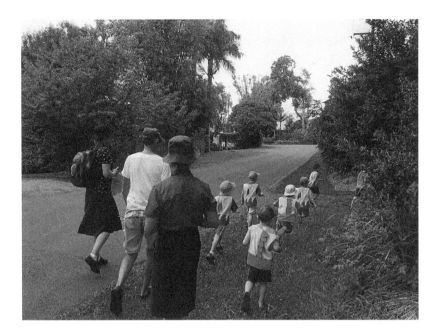

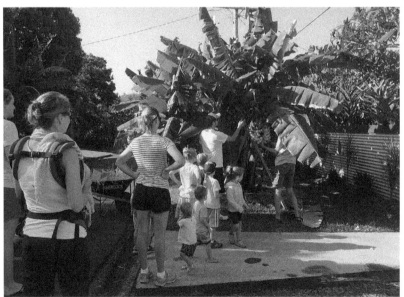

Figure 13.1a and b. The neighbourhood had become a vital component of the teaching program at the local childcare centre, Milford Lodge. Small groups would visit the streets to harvest fruit and vegetables, which were taken back to the centre and cooked. It was much loved by the children as a learning experience. Here they are visiting Clithro Avenue (top) and 'Banana Street' (Stephen Street; bottom). Photos courtesy of Caroline Kemp.

viable in all urban or suburban settings) the big picture benefits to our society are profound.

The benefits include the health credentials that are linked with positive connections, gentle exercise and a diet that is rich in fresh fruit and vegetables, all of which can assist with lowered rates of diabetes, cancer and heart disease. Advantages extend in all directions from reduced crime, due to what urban writer and activist Jane Jacobs terms 'eyes on the street' (the informal vigilance that comes with an active streetscape),[11] to the environmental advantages of cooler urban environments and 'improved' soil from composting, which sequesters more carbon and retains more life-sustaining water.

On another level are the benefits associated with inclusion of the elderly: passing of information and skills from one generation to another (gardening, preserving, cooking and fermenting), improved public space aesthetics and the sharing of neighbourhood resources such as lawn-mowers, swimming pools, gardening equipment and chicken tractors.[12]

Government-enforced rules and regulations dictate almost everything we do. Is spontaneity dead? Are we overly controlled by red tape? Have we lost the ability to critically and emphatically challenge, in real time, the problems that are generated by current planning and enforcement protocols? Faced with another form to fill out, another approval process and another permit, people disengage from the delights of the suburban everyday. Permits kill participation. They stop community from being our community. The stricter those rules associated with the approval process, the less neighbourly engagement takes place.

With a model, free from the constrictions of conventional organisational structure, and the restricting, conflicting, confusing demands and requirements of local government, participation was simple to generate. The three years from February 2014 until late 2016 saw exponential growth and enthusiasm.

However, this story of activating suburban public space through connection has a sour ending. In late November 2016, the families using the nature strip to grow fruit and vegetables were served a notice by the local council, adversarial in delivery, to cease action immediately. Put simply, 'planting, damaging or removing' any vegetation on council-controlled land was not allowed. According to a local bylaw, this activity required council permission. Based on the notice served on the fruit and vegetable growers of this precinct, thousands of families right across the municipality were in breach of this bylaw, through the action of planting vegetation on nature strips. Largely and some might say conveniently, these breaches went unnoticed.

Neighbourhood participation rates plummeted instantly, with roughly half the families served notice no longer interested in a project that was dictated by local government and encumbered by the associated costs of the municipality's requirement for permits and insurance (bearing in mind that, at the time the local municipality chopped and chipped those trees, they asserted that permits were free, but would not publically guarantee this status into the future). They opted to remove the food-producing nature strip gardens and return them to turf. What had taken eight years to germinate and grow through the production of fresh food – an active, cohesive and connected neighbourhood – was drastically reduced with further critical damage done when the council unashamedly chopped and chipped the precinct's beating heart, eighteen mature, fruit-laden citrus trees, early one morning in late May 2017. This action gained national attention and a focus on our local municipality, with community outcry from far and wide.

Design can connect people with their urban surrounds and to each other. For us, activation through food grown in the suburban environment was a means to disrupt the dominant suburban order while demonstrating the sheer productive capacity of Australia's vast tracts of suburban public places and spaces, particularly the nature strip. Society is in desperate need of place-specific solutions that are tailored to contemporary community need. In this context, perhaps the greatest lesson to be learnt from our story relates not only to the social and environmental sterility, austerity and inflexibility of the one-size-fits-all way in which public space risk is managed by local government, but also the propensity of some local governments to act with wilful disregard of the holistic good that is delivered to society through the activation of public space in this way.

PART 4

Multiple Pasts, Possible Futures?

Chapter 14

Learning from our Productive Past

Andrea Gaynor

Australian cities have long traditions of local food production. As such, they are a rich source of historical stories that can help us work toward more sustainable, resilient and fair food systems today. These stories point to the lost potential for local food production, as well as some of the risks and opportunities of regaining it. In tracing continuity and change over time, they also illuminate what is enduring and what is unique to our times. Without such guides, we are stuck with the narrow horizons and inexplicable profusion of the present.

I am poorly qualified to tell the oldest stories, as a *wadjela* whose family has lived on *Noongar Boodjar* for a scant few generations. As a historian, however, I know that Australian cities were founded on important sites for Indigenous food systems. The early colonists looked for places with sufficient fresh water and ports for shipping. The coastal, riparian and wetland plants and animals of these places had sustained local people for millennia, as part of complex and resilient food systems that combined cultivation and wild harvesting with land-management practices that put animals in particular places for hunting. Colonisation radically disrupted these practices, though they did not disappear overnight: Fanny Balbuk, born around the time Perth was founded, used to walk with her family from Matagarup (Heirisson Island) to Lake Kingsford, where she gathered gilgies (freshwater crayfish) and edible wetland plants. As the town of Perth developed, she continued to walk the same track, even breaking fences and forcing her way through a house built over the route. Lake Kingsford was drained for the construction of Perth train station and Balbuk died in 1907, amid a settler society that rejected most native foods.[1]

Colonists' ability to occupy Indigenous territory depended on the adaptability of their own food-producing plants and animals, which they kept close at hand in their burgeoning settlements. Melbourne's Fitzroy in the late-nineteenth century is an illustrative example. This municipality had experienced rapid growth from the beginning of the Victorian gold rush to the peak of Marvellous Melbourne's long boom. In 1891, it was home to 32,453 people, as well as a cacophony of productive animals: 131 cows, 42 goats, 149 turkeys and 18,000 fowls, in addition to 1614 horses. The residential areas to the east and south, with access to the open land around the Yarra River, were even more beastly.[2]

To contemporary urban agriculture enthusiasts, this image of late-nineteenth-century Fitzroy may appear arcadian, though it's important not to romanticise life in a city brimming with productive animals. There was conflict between neighbours over noise and smell. The flies that bred abundantly in poorly managed sties, stables and sheds might also carry deadly typhoid from the dunny to the table. Some animals were kept in woeful conditions with insufficient space, poor drainage and rotten food. Others, however, were loved as family members.[3] Many flourished – particularly in those urban centres, like Fremantle, that for many years retained a commonage on which stock could be grazed. Well-kept local animals produced fresh and nutritious milk, eggs and, occasionally, meat, as well as manure for gardens.[4]

While working families were the most likely to keep animals, many middle-class Melburnians with a little bit of space and security of tenure delighted in growing their own fruit and vegetables. Their reasons are familiar today: they liked the freshness and the flavour. As more men were employed in office jobs, they liked to get out of their suits and work up a sweat with a spade. Women tended tomatoes alongside toddlers and strengthened neighbourhood networks through exchange of produce. All debated whether growing your own food saved any money, though the expansion of food gardening in the Great Depression of the 1930s showed that a thrifty gardener could help keep food on the table.

Another element to the attractiveness of home food production was the symbolic independence it imparted. From the early days of colonisation, many free immigrants to Australia had been attracted by the idea that they could become independent on their own land. This desire underpinned the ill-fated push for closer settlement of rural Australia that emerged from the mid-nineteenth century, as well as the popularity of the suburban quarter-acre block with an extensive vegetable garden, fruit trees and maybe some poultry. This symbolic self-sufficiency didn't release (male) suburban food-producers from the need to seek an income elsewhere, but it allowed them to perform the ideals of 'manly independence' usually reserved for farmers.

A higher degree of food independence was required when the Second World War brought several threats to the Australian food system. After Japan entered the war, there was a shortage of agricultural inputs such as rubber and pesticides, as well as increased demand for exports to Britain and the need to feed service personnel stationed in the region. The national larder was looking too bare for comfort and greater self-provisioning was a means to fill the gap. It was also a home-front morale builder that had been employed to good effect in the UK and USA during World War I. From 1942, grassroots initiatives emerged first in the form of YWCA 'garden armies' that organised women to grow vegetables on land provided by local government and homeowners. Women in paid work volunteered on Saturday afternoons and homemakers volunteered during the week. School children, scouts and guides helped out at harvest time. Volunteers could buy the produce at a discounted rate and the proceeds went to the Australian Comforts Fund and Red Cross.

The Commonwealth Department of Commerce and Agriculture and state departments of agriculture followed in 1943, collaborating to launch a large-scale 'Grow Your Own' campaign targeting individual gardeners. Centred around patriotic messages in mass media, it used newspaper ads, radio broadcasts, posters, brochures and even stickers on gas and power bills to encourage households to grow their own vegetables and keep their own fowl (figure 14.1).

The Second World War food-production campaigns show us that it's possible to rapidly increase home food production in a crisis, but they also point to the kinds of difficulties that might be encountered. There were problems associated with the nationally coordinated campaign; for example, advice on vegetable growing was sometimes inappropriate for local conditions. The disruptions of war had also cut off the supply of gardening inputs like seeds, hoses and fertilisers, which limited the capacity for food production. Resources like open land and local manures were more available, however, than they are today. This probably enabled a fairly rapid increase in self-provisioning motivated by a sense of duty (and to some extent, need). After the crisis had subsided, however, and householders were no longer performing their loyalty in the vegetable patch, production declined: patriotism in war was no firm foundation on which to build a nation of urban farmers.

The conventional understanding is that after the war everyone got a car and a swimming pool and forgot about growing their own food – unless they had recently stepped off a boat from Italy or Yugoslavia. Certainly, many migrant families coming from rural Europe continued the production they had lived by until the disruption of war, though through the 1950s and '60s many Anglo-Australians also maintained at least a bit of food production, tucked away in spaces invisible to the street.

The 1970s saw somewhat of a revival of self-provisioning, as a new romanticism associated with the alternative lifestyles of the 1960s counterculture coincided with the oil shocks and stagflation that marked the end to the long post-war economic boom. In a volatile economic and political climate, many people grew their own food as a source of security and independence on the one hand, and reconnection with nature on the other. In the boom decade of the 1980s, home food production was also a way to be gourmet and to better the industrialised and tired produce from rapidly lengthening supply chains. In the 1990s, some saw it as a rehearsal for sustainable living. The desire for fresh and flavoursome food endured throughout, though the size of harvests was shrinking and most of the animals had been evicted.

LEARNING FROM OUR PRODUCTIVE PAST

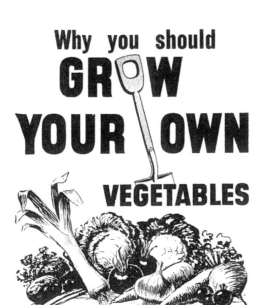

Figure 14.1. 'Grow Your Own' advertisement by the Commonwealth Department of Commerce and Agriculture, published in numerous Australian newspapers in August 1943.

Over the last 150 years, there has been a significant appetite for self-provisioning among Australian urban dwellers. To understand why it has decreased over time, we need to look less at motivation than at constraints. One of the earliest barriers was local government regulation of animals, driven by a particular vision of modern cities and suburbs under the guise of public health. These regulations disadvantaged those working-class and marginalised people who were most dependent on their animals: local government archives include heartbreaking letters from single mothers pleading to keep the goats that were their only means of providing milk for their children. Even today, many local governments retain regulations that make antiquated distinctions between 'farm' and 'pet' animals, and aim for prohibition rather than supporting sound management for sustainability, health and animal welfare.

Another important factor has been access to suitable land. As urban land has become more valuable and new lot sizes have reduced, an increasing number of people have started living in apartments and townhouses. Urban infill on the one hand, and the maturing urban forest on the other, have reduced the amount of suitable space for growing food at home in older suburbs. For many, self-provisioning on a substantial scale seems an unattainable dream.

Also crucial has been change in the organisation of labour and people's use of time. The work of food production in Anglo-Australian households was often shared between men and women – though of course many households of 'maiden aunts' or bachelors and their same-sex companions grew food too. In more conventional homes, men in paid work were usually responsible for the heavy physical labour of vegetable-bed preparation, while female homemakers (and often children) would undertake the daily maintenance of poultry and vegetables. As more women entered the paid workforce during the post-war economic boom (and achieved a degree of economic independence), many households found themselves with insufficient time to devote to the planning and upkeep that traditional self-provisioning requires.

This era saw a gathering intensification of capitalist colonisation of the world, in which goods and services previously produced in the home – food, child care, maintenance, entertainment – were increasingly commodified and subject to market relations. Planning and local government regulation reinforced the status of residential suburbs as sites of consumption. In this context, self-provisioning on a significant scale became more difficult but retained its important symbolic dimensions, not least as a declaration of (potential) independence from the long and vulnerable supply chains of big retail.

This short and partial history of Australian urban productive landscapes highlights the extent to which non-commercial production was undertaken by individual households on private property. As such, it was contingent on the theft of land from Indigenous people and its reconfiguration as private property. The beneficiaries – settler land owners and (less often) tenants – valued this land and often used it ingeniously for productive purposes, though rarely in any coordinated or collaborative way.

While first Indigenous places, then public spaces have been engrossed by private property and commercial interests over time, the self-provisioning story includes a long tradition of resistance to such urban enclosure, particularly among working-class people. From house cows grazed along river frontages and town commons in the late-nineteenth century, to backyard bees foraging in local gardens in the early twenty-first century, people have used urban livestock to appropriate urban spaces for production. Wild harvesting of fish in rivers and foraging of overhanging fruit and nuts have also confounded the enclosure of urban food. Over time, such productive uses were often regulated – sometimes wisely – or discouraged, though never entirely eliminated.

From vertical gardens to wicking beds, self-provisioning remains a site of innovation and potential to contribute to more resilient and sustainable food systems in our burgeoning cities. However, history shows us that it is not the only answer. Self-provisioning historically helped reduce urban inequality to a degree, though its potential here was limited: the urban poor could always have benefited from more self-supplied food, but due to lack of space, lack of access to appropriate and secure land, lack of skills and support, and regulations prohibiting animal-keeping, they have been least empowered to get it.

One of the distinctive features of the 'revival' of urban food production in recent decades is a growing attention to the more communal dimensions of food production, moving beyond a self-provisioning focus to encompass food production as a means of strengthening community and providing fresh and nutritious food to those least able to acquire it by other means. In a context of growing precarity and disenchantment with the exclusiveness of commodified urban space, as well as the growing problem of food desertification (diminishing access to fresh and healthy food, especially in less-well-off areas), these are important experiments in sustaining non-proprietorial, just and nourished worlds.

Chapter 15

Feeding Melbourne: Market Gardening in the Sandbelt: 1950s–1970s

Liz Clay

The freshly dug soil just had to be run across. My unshod feet were unable to withstand the scorching heat of the tiny grains of silica exposed to the summer heat. To avoid burnt feet as I ran, I would spear my toes through the layer of hot sand into the cool, moist subsoil below – quite exhilarating and something I would love to do over and over again.

My job was to get the afternoon tea for the 'boys', a generic term used by my mother to describe my brothers Warwick and Roger, my Dad and any other bloke that happened to be around. I was typically the only female of the species to be found out in the paddocks, scratching around in the soil with the others.

As a twelve year old I was probably a bit young to help with the loading, although I had just spent the afternoon with the team picking up spuds. I was therefore elected to drive the truck along the empty rows while the boys loaded the hessian bags onto the tray – those spuds heading to a merchant probably ended up as potato cakes or chips for a string of fish-and-chip shops in suburban Melbourne.

Places where I grew up, played and worked with my family on our 48-acre market garden are now gone – unrecognisable with the concrete, tar and bricks well established in the landscape. The houses and footpaths of the south eastern suburbs have for decades replaced the once familiar dark grey soils where neat rows of vegetables grew topped and tailed by a matrix of headlands. Those headlands allowed the movement of tractors and workers to tend and harvest the wide range of vegetables that fed Melbourne from the early 1950s through to the 1980s, after which the veggies made way for the bulldozers and cement trucks.

The following is a very short account of my experiences as a young girl and teen growing up in a market gardening community on the sandbelt in south east Melbourne during the late 1950s through to the early '70s. A decade on from the end of the Second World War, it was an interesting time of urban expansion, immigration, then to conscription and the Vietnam War via Women's Lib and rock and roll. Many of these political and social issues were of little real interest to my conservative farming family. Nevertheless, we were touched by all of them in one way or another and, as my father would often say, whatever was going on in the world '…people still got to eat'.

The sandbelt is richly significant – a geological feature stretching from Brighton, Bentleigh, Moorabbin, Heatherton, Keysborough through to Cranbourne, Devon Meadows and the Mornington Peninsula. The reach of this soil type determined the siting and path of expansion for market gardening families who made up a discrete community involved in growing fresh produce over the last 100 years.

My story coincides with a wave of vegetable farmer migration. The second generation of those who had first gardened in the Bentleigh/Moorabbin area bought new land. My dad Fred (Freddie) Clay and mother Joyce moved to Keysborough from Moorabbin soon after they were married in 1950. They, and many others, left behind farms that had produced the great majority of Melbourne's fresh food and were now being developed to house the expanding population of postwar Melbourne. Indeed, like the sandbelt itself, this migration was to happen again as the next generation of veggie growers in the '80s uprooted and followed it across the landscape. They moved out to Cranbourne and the Mornington Peninsula, the pavement of the urban sprawl at their heels.

As a very little child, the early days for me at Keysborough involved exploring the little green-hooded orchids, mossy logs and fungi amongst the bracken ferns and lonely stringybarks, trees of the remnant roadside vegetation. Networks of drains were established across the district by gardeners to increase the water runoff through the thick band of sandy clay loam topsoil that was met abruptly by strong clay subsoils. The topsoils were perfect for gardening, as they themselves were very well drained, allowing growers to return to the paddock with their tractors and work the ground soon after any rain event. This allowed veggie growing all year round. The agricultural pipes and drains were there to deal with those impenetrable clay subsoils and emptied their contents into lower-lying properties sacrificed to salt and water logging, which were used to run a few kids' ponies.

Our adjoining low-lying paddocks suffered the same fate. Here lived retired Roany, Freddie's old draught horse from the Moorabbin years. Roany had once pulled the dray, loaded with veggies, along steel tram tracks to the Vic Market in Melbourne. Freddie wasn't much of a horseman. He was quick to take up the new technologies of the day, which Massey Ferguson and International Harvester were bringing onto the market. A much-admired red Dodge truck joined the fleet and replaced Roany.

Story has it that Freddie and Joyce were able to develop and pay for the farm's irrigation infrastructure and drainage, buy machinery and build a brand-new cream brick veneer house in the fashion of the day in the first two years after arriving at Keysborough. As fresh food remained in short supply in the early '50s, the first crop of potatoes and cabbages fetched enormous prices even by today's standard. One guinea for a dozen cabbages or a bushel bag of potatoes was very good money. Those impressive yields, gained from the accumulated nutrition of soils previously under pasture for years, gave us good fortune and set solid foundations for our family for the next twenty-five years.

Getting the load up for market was an all-day affair, with all hands on deck. The biggest market of the week was Monday morning, so Sunday was never a day of rest. Without cool storage, produce had to be picked and packed in an orderly fashion with wet hessian bags covering produce that needed to stay cool and moist. Our main shed

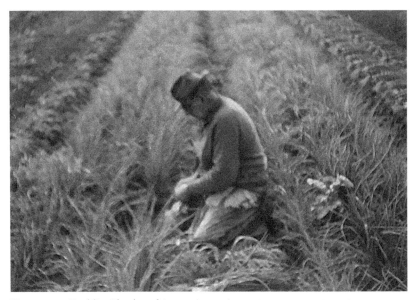

Figure 15.1. Freddie Clay bunching spring onions. Photo courtesy of Liz Clay.

was a big old wooden barn with a high gable roof containing a loft. The space was open either end creating a breezeway with adjoining bays on either side. Mature macrocarpa cypress trees had been planted close to the north keeping the whole area reasonably well protected from the sun.

At one end of one of the bays was a locked shed reeking of all sorts of familiar smells from the acrid chemicals that caused the district to stink from time to time, to the tins of seed and the reefs of parsnip seeds hanging from the rafters drying on the stalk. All sorts of stuff was kept there: rolls of hemp string for bunching, net bags for onions, stacks of hessian potato bags, nails, hand tools including a class set of weeding implements and a range of hoes – dutch hoes, stirrup hoes, chip hoes then garden forks, spades and the intimidating cabbage choppers.

Just to the east of the main shed was a persistent rambling blackberry bush that hid a derelict old well and the entrance to another tin shed partly squashed by a limb from one of the cypress trees. One had to negotiate the plank dropped across a drain and steady yourself using the trunk of the tree to access this gloomy little shed that contained all things irrigation. Nearby was the carrot washer.

We used to love getting into the carrot washer – a huge drum made of wooden slats lined with water jets attached to an internal pipe in the centre of the drum. This would pressure-wash the carrots, parsnips or any other root crop that could handle the rough and tumble of the rotating drum, which was powered through the drive shaft of the tractor and geared to allow turning by hand. As kids, we would take turns to be a carrot locked into the barrel while the others rocked the thing backwards and forwards. Luckily, it took a lot of effort to turn it over so there was no great risk of children being tumbled. The only real downside was the potential of being left locked in the washer as siblings ran off smitten by the cleverness of their cruel joke.

Help on the farm was necessary and for as long as I can remember the 'old place', the old homestead across the yard from the shed, housed a series of Dutch foremen and their families. The wave of migrants in the '60s and '70s provided opportunities to employ some wonderfully experienced farmers from Europe to help on the farm. Morry, our first employee, was also an experienced horseman who soon became a very competent ploughman with the tractor. We employed Italian and Greek workers during key harvest times, a number of whom worked hard with their extended families to buy their own plots of land to garden or become vegetable merchants. I recall teams of 'white' Russians employed through semi-organised labour-hire outfits to harvest crops. Men, women and children arrived in packed cars, all pitching in during the long hot days. My guess the reference to 'white' Russians was to do with their resistance to communist rule making them clearly more acceptable than those branded 'red'!

Homeless man Laurie, from another market gardening family, lived with us for a while. He had been in a motorbike accident and the resulting head injuries left him with a form of epilepsy. Nevertheless, Laurie was a handy bloke to have around. With his grey 'Fergie' tractor, he worked for numerous farmers as a ploughman and was well recognised for his prowess in creating straight rows.

Keeping that beautiful sandy loam in good condition was always going to be a challenge. Sandy soils need a drip feed of nutrients and constant supply of organic matter to keep the nutrients from leaching away. There is not much grace, so little and often is the rule even in the good loamy soils. Some soluble fertilisers available in convenient bags were used but they had the tendency to leach through the soil profile before the crop had time to use it up. Freddie preferred local inputs.

At the back of the property was an egg farm – rows of sheds where caged birds were housed. From time to time, dry chicken manure was collected. The tractor and trailer were used to load, pick up and spread it all within the course of one afternoon. I considered the only thing worse than being the tractor driver when the wind was blowing was being one of my brothers shovelling off the dry shit and accidently discovering an ancient egg in the process. The utterings of disgust were understandable.

Freddie would also bring loads of stable manure from the racing stables at Mentone on the way home from market. The stable manure was put straight onto the waiting soil ready to be ploughed in – it was rarely composted, although occasionally I would admire the steam issuing from a random heap on a frosty winter's morning. The straw drenched in urine and peppered with golden pebbles of poo was a lovely feed for the microbes in the soil. I wonder if Freddie realised it was the soil ecosystems he was feeding – all those little organisms breaking down that stable material, providing nutrients to the plants. I reckon he probably had some idea, despite the fact the agronomy of the day was well and truly promoting the use of chemically derived fertilisers and agricultural chemicals. He knew some of those inputs used in agriculture were toxic.

It was instilled into us to wash any fruit that was brought home from the market. Apples and cherries were singled out for special attention. He wasn't so adamant about our own veggies, which we would pluck, clean the soil off on our clothes and munch on as we walked across the paddocks. I confess to devouring many a carrot or burying my face in a massive juicy turnip as I headed to the horse paddock – mmm…delicious! My Shetland pony Blacky never missed an opportunity to snatch the heads of lettuce if I wasn't watching when I rode around the farm.

As a little kid, I would sometimes accompany Freddie, trotting along in my gumboots to keep up with his stride. Used to walking the paddock alone, he would use my company as an opportunity to provide a running commentary of what was going on with the crops.

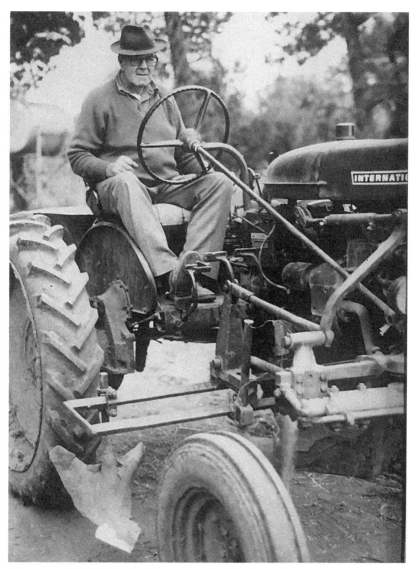

Figure 15.2. Freddie Clay heading out to do a bit of weeding. Photo courtesy of Liz Clay.

To a rhythmical stride, perhaps even a march looking left then right observing any changes, I recall him explaining variations in the crops – why some plants were not doing so well because the sprinkler hadn't reached them or the manure wasn't spread evenly or weeds were taking hold. On one of these excursions, he stopped mid-stride, sunk to his knees and drove his hands into the soil extracting a handful, then he sniffed it and poked it under my nose uttering, 'Look! You could eat this stuff!' I had no idea what he was talking about and thought his suggestion a little odd, but his actions and those words remain etched into my memory.

Big brother Warwick reckons Freddie, although an admired grower of quality produce, was never as progressive or as quick to pick up on new technologies as some of our younger neighbours. Irrigation was a good case in point. Whilst we were dragging around hoses and scratching in the soil to attach them to underground taps, the Corrigans next door and the Andrews across the road had lovely grids of permanent sprinklers painted white so that no one would run over them – something that even Laurie would do from time to time on our place. Those innovations meant a line of sprinklers could be turned on from one gate valve and would have saved us a lot of time and money.

Another enviable advancement that we did not have were turkey nest dams. Once again, our neighbours had these. Turkey nest dams captured runoff water from the paddocks, collected water from roadsides and saved winter rains – all for summer irrigation. Our crops were irrigated from the mains water supply courtesy of the Yarra River via the Melbourne Metropolitan Board of Works. I can remember the stress the water bills created for my parents, particularly at the time when the 'Board' was preparing for the extensive expansion of Melbourne's water infrastructure in the late '60s. Freddie persevered for a short time with skyrocketing bills after the plans for the Dingley bypass road were released that would have seen our farm split in two. It proposed a 10-acre corridor through the middle of our property, to be compulsorily acquired at some future date for a freeway.[1]

That was the last straw. It was clear the viability of the farm at Keysborough was under question and plans to move the operation further afield were set in place.

Freddie first rented, then finally bought, land at Barham in NSW; my seventeen-year-old brother, Warwick, was sent up there to work on the property while the Keysborough farm was slowly wound down and eventually sold to developers.

For years, the land where we had once farmed hosted empty weeds in the place where vegetables once grew. The 'old place', long without any inhabitants, slowly collapsed, then finally burned to the ground – the work of arsonists. At last the bulldozers arrived to create a huge hole and the lovely old sheds and trees were pushed up, burned and buried. It did not take long to erase all traces of the past, including the old well, revealed for brief moment during the levelling.

The land that once grew food to sustain a population was being prepared for other human endeavours. When it comes to food and food production, the soil is hero. Freddie understood this. The fundamental basis of growing healthy food is the health of the soil. The soil that is not dirt, not an inert substrate, but a thriving ecosystem of millions of living organisms confounding in the processes it can perform subject to our care and respect.

In a continent with such precious little good soil for growing food, we are witnessing the loss of our productive agricultural land to competing uses. The sandbelt – a recognised feature of Melbourne's landscape that fed our city for the last 100 years – is uttering its last gasps, forever lost to the appetite of its sprawling suburbs. A generation on, the last of the market gardening families I grew up with, now farming at Cranbourne, hang on while the sandy loams now grow houses around them.

My family no longer farms – it's just me who scratches around in the soil on my own little farm in Gippsland. I grow my veggies to organic standards in a polyculture of fruit and nut trees and take my harvest to farmers markets in Melbourne each week. My upbringing at Keysborough and Freddie's passion for the soil have been my foundation – and I'm still loving that warm earth under my feet.

Chapter 16

Australia, 1945: The Future Begins

Srebrenka Kunek and John Shone

The street
>   filled with tomatoes,
>   midday,
>   summer,
>   light is
>   halved
>   like
>   a
>   tomato,
>   its juice
>   runs
>   through the streets

From 'Ode to Tomatoes', by Pablo Neruda[1]

Part 1: History speaks

To know your history is to have insight into your future, or, 'When is a tomato more than what you eat?' We address this question by presenting the nexus between Australian Federal Government post–World War II immigration policies and programs and arable agricultural food producing land in peri-urban areas, up to today.

This chapter encompasses Australia as a whole, with specific reference to Melbourne. This is due to Melbourne being the nation's manufacturing capital in the postwar period until the beginning of the 1980s, which has had particular implications for food-producing agricultural land today and into the future.

In 1945, Australia changed forever. Towards the end of World War II in the Pacific, Arthur Calwell, Labor MP and future Federal Minister for Immigration, spoke in Parliament of the immigration of foreigners and border security, in the same breath. Ironically, Calwell, like the majority of Australian politicians and indeed Australians of the time, was a staunch believer in, and defender of, the White Australia policy, according to which, the nation was defined as a white and British country. On 2 August 1945, he defined immigration as 'our second chance to survive' due to the need for increased population and expansion of the economy.[2] It was, he said, a matter of 'populate or perish', in reference to what was seen as the near-inevitability of a future Asian takeover of an under-populated land after the near-miss with Japan in World War II.

While the subject is far greater than the statistics, they are indicative. Australia at the beginning of the twentieth century was 98 per cent British.[3] In 1947, people of non-English-speaking background were 10 per cent of the Australian population, rising to 22 per cent by the mid 1970s and to 28 per cent by 2014, predicted to rise further in the coming decades.[4] The ethnic composition of Australia has changed dramatically in the last 100 years, with profound (and we believe fundamentally positive) consequences for the polity and society as a whole.

We present federal government immigration policies and programs that have driven this transformation from the perspective of housing, food and the role of arable agricultural land in Melbourne, as we comment on urban agriculture.[5]

Part 2: Three historical periods and the birth of urban sprawl

From 1945 to the end of the 1960s was the period of federal government reconstruction aimed at the delivery of the new 'Australian Way of Life' of higher living standards, income security, housing and opportunity for all following the widespread austerity measures during the war – including, as Andrea Gaynor discusses in chapter 14, the 'Grow Your Own' home gardening campaign.

The southern European immigration programs were pivotal to this new idea of the nation, operating based on concepts of race and racial preference for northern European and British migrant families. The Southern European program (1951 to 1969) was designed to function as a 'tap' of females (defined as consumers) and males (defined as producers), but not both together as families.[6] The program was key to federal government management of economic development for increasing the Australian-born birth rate, central to the new Australia.[7]

Melbourne became the migrant capital and the manufacturing hub, a flow on from the role of the city during World War II. However, the shortage of housing, due to the lack of all forms of building materials, presented a challenge for the planned population growth. It was also a highly charged social and political issue known to be affecting low-income and middle-class Australians.[8] Melbourne was in a unique position to solve this problem: the city had cheap inner-urban housing and a supply of even cheaper arable agricultural food-producing land on the outskirts.[9]

The result was the urban sprawl that continues today. It was a choice made by the state government then, and one it continues to make now. Urban sprawl was a direct outcome of federal and state government economic development and planning policies in the postwar period. Today, we still have a pressing need for affordable housing, which is more acute than it has ever been. However, the unfortunate impact of urban sprawl is that, as we have seen with the experience of Liz Clay and her family in the previous chapter, it results in the continued loss of peri-urban farmland, which is seriously compromising our food security and food sovereignty.

Knowing our history empowers us to redirect these historical forces for the establishment of an economy based on food production and to address housing affordability.

The 1970s to the end of the 1990s marked the end of post-war economic growth. The period was defined by domestic economic instability within a global context in the 1970s of rising inflation and unemployment (stagflation) and three major Australian economic recessions in 1974–75, 1982–83 and 1990–91.[10] This period was also defined by a shift to Asian migration with the abandonment of the White Australia policy by the Holt Liberal government in 1966[11] and its formal legal cessation in 1973 under the Whitlam government.[12]

Below, we examine the nexus between immigration and agricultural land in peri-urban areas around Melbourne, the major shifts in the idea of Australia as a nation being a 'lucky country' to today, with the shadow of growing food insecurity.[13]

Part 3: Post-war reconstruction to the end of the 1960s
In 1945, the federal and state governments were set to deliver: homes, civic infrastructure, employment, social protection, a higher standard of living and a new Australian Way of Life, prosperous and abundant. There was the confidence, mandate and experience of directing the economy and country after winning the war, which government planners applied to reconstruction.[14] Their decision making was also informed by their knowledge of pre-war Australia: the shortage of housing, low birth rates from the beginning of the nineteenth century, the 1930s Depression and high unemployment.[15]

The critical issue addressed by reconstruction planners through postwar immigration was the need to provide an immediate supply of young adults without increasing demand on goods and services. The 'Australian Way' was both an economic and political need.[16] The delivery of this 'Way of Life' also represented its counterpart: the danger of inflation that 'dominated' federal government according to Treasurer Ben Chifley.[17]

The government mechanisms for controlling these conditions to deliver planned outcomes varied according to their political brand. The Labor government, advised by the Keynesian John Dedman, was about control over production and consumption, financed by taxation and borrowings.[18] The long Liberal era under Robert Menzies (1949–66) saw a shift to resources, namely government deployment of men and materials.[19] Government management of population types and numbers, through the lever of non-British immigration, was a key tool to deliver the new Australia. The shadow side of this model and its implementation was the Southern European program, together with the loss of arable agricultural land.

Basic industries, production of goods and services, housing and public works were required to address low natural (i.e. Australian-born) population increases,[20] a continuing subject of government concern in the postwar period.[21] W. D. Borrie, the prominent demographer and adviser to government, advocated for conditions 'favourable to fertility' in his 1958 book, *The Peopling of Australia*.[22]

For the first time in Australian history, immigration was based on economic planning of population growth (defined as 2 per cent), with immigration making up a 1 per cent per annum increase of the total population.[23] The less racially 'desirable' southern Europeans provided government planners with control over gender, numbers and race intakes and the regulation of monthly entry for economic management purposes.

How? Firstly, they provided a supply of labour, male and female, for deployment to essential industries and public works under a two-year contract.[24] Secondly, gender selection targeted men as producers and women as consumers, specifically through the assisted-passage program operating until the end of the 1960s. The program was turned on and off based on economic planning and was instrumental in managing the 'genie' of inflation through regulating consumption and production. It was central to managing the recessions of 1951–52, 1955–56[25] and 1960–61, until the supply of migrant labour dwindled due to improved economic conditions in Europe.[26]

Part 4: Agricultural land, manufacturing and Melbourne

The significant role of the postwar southern European immigration program needs to be viewed together with another startling historical fact.

Agriculture and farm production were not expanded as part of reconstruction planning, despite requests for food exports from Britain[27] and government planners knowing that farmers lacked materials and equipment. Their needs were ignored.[28] A significant publication of the time states that agricultural producers' expectations were that 'men would come back to farming from the forces and the munition factories' and there would be 'materials for replacement and repair'; their 'disillusionment [on being ignored] was bitter'.[29] The emphasis of reconstruction policy was on manufacturing, which accounted for 25 per cent of national employment, with agriculture making up less than 10 per cent of jobs.[30] Melbourne was the centre of manufacturing growth with a focus on the expanding automotive industry.[31]

We are dealing with a significant lost opportunity. In 1945, government planning and implementation of the new Australia came at the expense not only of southern European families, but also of agriculture, food production and a more diversified manufacturing sector. Victoria's regional centres, supported by rail networks from the 1870s, provided a viable solution for preserving prime food-producing land. The opportunity to couple food production with food processing as the basis of the Victorian economy post–World War II was there, yet the weight of government policy was thrown behind the automotive sector. But the opportunity to support food processing remains an option that can be legislated for today.

Former agricultural land served, of course, another purpose. Subdivided, former food-producing agricultural land fuelled the housing and development industry, a trend with which we are all too familiar. We could, however, have followed a different path: the so-called Viennese model – in particular the transformative era of 'Red Vienna' (1919–43) – rather than the Californian model of endless urban sprawl and choking freeways.[32] Apartment housing around urban railway stations, evidenced belatedly since the 1990s, could have been the policy directive applied to regional centres post–World War II, resulting in a very different reality of urban planning and food sovereignty.

The natural increase of the Australian-born population, including growing numbers resulting from inter-marriage amongst the 'new' and 'old' Australians, continued to rise after 1945 through the 1950s and the following decade.[33] With the dream of home ownership actively promoted as integral to the 'Australian Way of Life', Australian-born families purchased large houses in the outer suburbs newly created by the subdivision of former agricultural food-producing land. Home ownership surged from 50 per cent at the end of the war to 70 per cent in the early 1960s.[34] Everyone embraced the dream: by 1981, non-Australian-born home ownership was above the 70 per cent figure for the Australian born.[35] And for government planners and politicians, it worked: the Australian economy grew faster than other developed nations in the 1950s to 1960s within the context of global economic stability.[36]

Part 5: Our heritage: Srebrenka Kunek and John Shone

During this period, an alternative non-manufacturing production was taking place, led by southern European migrant families employing the 'garden' method of agriculture, meaning 'the cultivation of small plots of annual crops' of significance to the life of smaller towns.[37] This sounds very much like the concept of urban villages today.[38]

Our family's migration was due to us being members of the Croatian Peasant Party, outlawed due to its opposition to the Nazi Third Reich occupiers of Croatia during World War II. After 1945, under the Yugoslav regime, the party went underground and operated abroad due to its support for peasant farmers on arable peri-urban land and in agricultural areas, and for being pro-democracy.

The practice of backyard food growing was also part of life in the western suburbs of Melbourne. In 1953, John (aged three), lived on three farms, all integrated for food production. North Cundare was the dairy farm and Yat Nat the homestead at Balmoral. Number 93 Summerhill Road, West Footscray, was a poultry farm with associated workshops and food gardens owned by Great Aunt Flo Linquist. She took on the Victorian Egg Board in the 1960s, fighting for the right for citizens to have poultry in urban backyards. In 1954, John (aged four) moved to Hex Street, Tottenham, where all fifty-nine houses had vegetable gardens and fifty-nine different languages were spoken.

We have replicated aspects of our heritage in our cultural-development professional practice, as evidenced in Taradale Food Gardens co-farming project and the installation *Navigating the Victorian Ethnic Food Trail,* 1996.[39] As Victorians, we have a powerful heritage of agriculture and food production in the peri-urban and rural areas. However, federal and state government policies have for decades

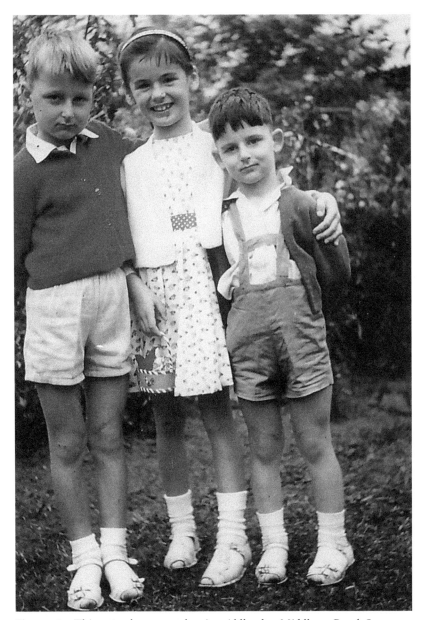

Figure 16.1. This 1960 photo was taken in middle-class Middlesex Road, Surrey Hills, the first home of the extended Kunek family. I am standing in the middle with my cousins Tom (left) and Paul (right). In the background, you can just see a tomato on an expansive tomato bush. We left our CBD apartment in Zagreb, Croatia, and migrated to Melbourne between 1954 and 1959. Our grandmother Marija Kunek turned the back garden into a high-yield food bowl. Photo courtesy of Srebrenka Kunek.

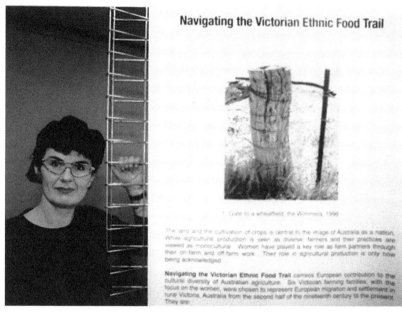

Figure 16.2. Dr Srebrenka Kunek, Navigating the Victorian Ethnic Food Trail, installation, Shepparton Art Gallery, Victoria, 1998. Photo courtesy of Srebrenka Kunek and John Shone.

favoured export farming over small-scale intensive food enterprises focused on domestic food security. Using our collective heritage and current knowledge, we can transition into a vibrant food economy supporting populations in smart regional catchments, serviced by trains and freight, delivering premium quality food to domestic and global markets.

Our food heritage includes Irish-born potato farmers in the Warrnambool and Port Fairy areas and Ballarat.[40] From the mid-nineteenth century, Scandinavians, Danes, Norwegians and Finns settled on farms. Swiss nationals settled in the La Trobe Valley establishing vineyards.[41] German farmers settled in the Wimmera, Western Victoria, and in the outskirts of Melbourne in the mid- to late-nineteenth century.[42] Asian market gardens flourished up to the introduction of the infamous White Australia policy.

In the post–World War II period, Italians farmed in the Ovens Valley and Greeks from Macedonia in Shepparton.[43] In 1947, the majority of Croatians, Italians and Greeks worked in agriculture.[44] At the beginning of the 1970s, the Dutch had the highest percentage of farmers in terms of the total workforce of Dutch origin, establishing dairy farming in Gippsland.[45]

Part 6: 1970s to the end of the 1990s

At the end of the 1960s, the ready supply of southern European migrants ceased due to improved economic conditions in Europe. Australian immigration selection policies were no longer part of economic planning of population management, thus marking the end of the application of the Keynesian model by government economic planners.[46] Quotas became the focus of the program.[47]

In the 1970s and 1980s, the global economy became 'unstable' and Australia experienced three major recessions. In 1983, the Hawke–Keating government removed industry tariffs and wage protections introduced by John Curtin,[48] representing the end of manufacturing and the introduction of the 'open economy' in the era of globalisation.[49]

Migration, which had had bipartisan support, became a political issue from the beginning of the 1970s, and is still a major feature of the current political context. Following the abandonment of the White Australia policy, the 1970s was a period of Asian migration, with the 1980s being a period of record Chinese migration. The Keating government introduced the skilled migration program in 1990–91, continued by John Howard from 1996. The first quarter of the twenty-first century has been dominated by Asian and Indian education migration, leading to the higher education sector becoming Australia's third-largest earner of export revenue, behind iron and coal.[50]

Part 7: First quarter of the twenty-first century and into the future

The distinguishing feature of the Australian Government's immigration program from the 1970s through the first quarter of the twenty-first century is economic development based on population growth through migration.[51]

The prominent economist Saul Eslake comments on economic growth based only on population growth as 'not worth having as it is not improving people's living conditions'. The trend is set to continue, with Melbourne's population predicted to increase to at least eight million by 2050, according to census figures.[52] In 2017, economists stated that new housing construction in Melbourne and Sydney had grown strongly since 2013, relative to public investment, which has been 'flat' in all states for several years.[53]

With an estimated eight million people by 2050, Melbourne will require at least 60 per cent more food than we are able to deliver today. Based on the current growth of the built environment of Melbourne, food-producing capacity is estimated to fall to around 18 per cent, due to population growth and urban sprawl.[54]

But here's the sting: state government revenues flow from new settler arrivals and housing in the form of state-derived tax from property taxes. The outcome is that land tax and stamp duty have risen by over 80 per cent in the last five years.[55]

We are witnesses of the major transition from affordable homes, abundant food and a healthy lifestyle being central to the idea of Australia as a nation, to affordable housing and food not being a reality for all citizens.[56]

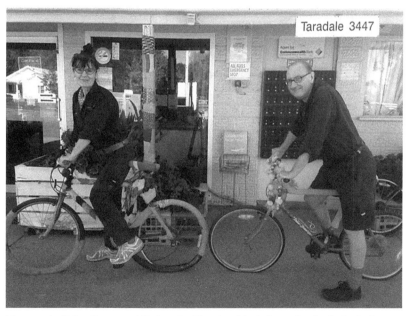

Figure 16.3. John Shone and Srebrenka Kunek with their garden beds (inclusive of tomatoes) at the Goods Shed, Taradale, Central Victoria, 2016. Photo courtesy of Srebrenka Kunek and John Shone.

Concluding remarks

When is growing a Pablo Neruda tomato a political act? When we grow food with the awareness of our agricultural and food-producing history, heritage and capacity for change.

Today, we have sound role models and urban village examples. What has been, can be reinvented, even at a petrol station, as seen in the photo of John and Srebrenka.

Our history speaks to us today and into the future.

Conclusion

Laying the Foundations for Sustainable Urban Food Systems in Australia

Nick Rose

As the various contributors to this anthology have affirmed, manifestations of what many regard as a generalised twenty-first-century crisis for humanity are especially acute in the life-giving field of agriculture and food. Speaking in terms of political economy, contemporary food systems in Australia (and globally) are accurately categorised as being oligopolistic: they are dominated by a handful of powerful agri-chemical, grain- and meat-packaging and trading, food-and-beverage-processing and supermarket corporations.[1] In recent decades, and reflective of a profound trajectory towards what Andrea described in chapter 14 as the increasing commodification of life, the driving imperative of these corporate actors has been profit maximisation and the generation of shareholder returns.[2] In this, they have been very successful. Agri-food production and retailing, and allied industries, are highly profitable.[3] The dominant agri-food corporations and their peak bodies have also been very successful in working with major political parties and government departments to erect a legal and fiscal architecture that is favourable to the expansion of the status quo.

There is, however, a great contradiction at the heart of national and global food systems. While these systems currently generate substantial profits for agri-food corporations and generous dividends for their shareholders, they also produce very poor outcomes for human health and wellbeing, as well as highly destructive environmental impacts. By some estimates, as many as two billion people are malnourished or undernourished, whilst a further 750 million are obese with more than one billion at risk of obesity.[4] In 2017, researchers calculated the total human health cost of food systems at US$13 trillion or one-sixth of global GDP.[5] Agri-food systems are leading generators of greenhouse-gas emissions and land-use change and, therefore, are major drivers of biodiversity loss.[6]

A recent assessment of the total value of ecosystem services estimated their value at US$125 trillion. Such services contribute significantly more to human well-being than global GDP. Further research found that the loss of such services due to land-use change (not including climate change, the use of agrichemicals or other human activities) can be estimated in the range of US$4.3 to US$20.2 trillion per year.[7] We can reasonably assume, given the scale of the land-clearing practices that convert native forest and grasslands to vast industrialised monocultures, that current global agri-food systems are responsible for a significant proportion of the loss of these invaluable ecosystem services.[8] These statistics – and they are but a mere handful of those that could be cited – are reflective of what Katherine Gibson evocatively termed the 'history of *uncommoning*' that has accompanied the era of the Great Acceleration.[9]

While these losses and costs are regarded as 'externalities' by agri-food corporations and traders in commodity markets, such an accounting sleight of hand will merely delay the day of ecological reckoning. The current dominant industrial food system – and, by implication, the current economic paradigm of which it forms an essential part – is undermining the health and well-being of substantial and growing human and non-human populations and, at the same time, the integrity of local, regional and global ecosystems and climatic stability. By so doing, it is encountering its own biophysical contradictions: it is undermining the conditions of its own reproduction.[10] It is thus, not only destructive but *self-destructive* and unsustainable by definition.

CONCLUSION

This is what the authors of the 2017 report published by the International Panel of Experts on Sustainable Food Systems captured in the title *Too Big to Feed,* and further in the report's key message:

> *Dominant firms have become too big to feed humanity sustainably, too big to operate on equitable terms with other food system actors, and too big to drive the types of innovation we need.* [11]

The authors identified eight systemic 'lock-ins' that constitute barriers to change, as well as several key strategies to begin to cut through these lock-ins (see figure 17.1).

The case for transformative change is overwhelming and urgent. The choices made in previous decades, as documented by IPES-Food at the global level and as shown in the Melbourne context in chapter 16 by Srebrenka Kunek and John Shone, have led us to a present of seemingly endless urban sprawl, the loss of rich soils and housing unaffordability for growing numbers of people. Further, as

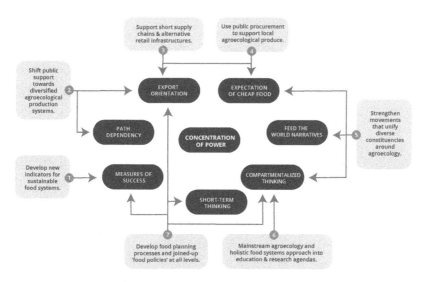

Figure 17.1. IPES-Food: Turning industrial food system lock-ins into entry points for change. Image courtesy of IPES-Food.

the history of market gardening in Keysborough in Melbourne's sandbelt narrated by Liz Clay (chapter 15) demonstrates, those choices and the urban development dynamics that they at first promoted and then embedded have also led to the loss of food sovereignty, growing dependence on imported food and the prospect of rising food prices and food insecurity.

A time of great change is upon us, whether we are ready or not. The choices and actions we take now will be what shape the coming decades and the contours of life for future generations. Multiple struggles over what the future can and should be have been underway for many years. These struggles are intensifying in the face of accelerating climatic, financial and geopolitical instability. Manifestations of a generalised political crisis can be seen in the sharp swing to the far right in the United States with the election in 2016 of Donald Trump and his brand of defensive, ultra-nationalistic and openly racist, anti-immigrant politics. For David Holmgren (chapter 7), times of growing crisis portend a resurgence of non-monetary gift and sharing economies that he captures so well through multiple case studies in his latest book, *RetroSuburbia*. As regards the continued flourishing of what Holmgren terms 'garden farming' and the associated practices of household and community non-monetary economies, for him it is a question of whether these 'go viral' or 'retreat to enclaves in the shadows of an increasingly armoured and centralised economy'.

This is not idle speculation. The policies and laws, as well as the technologies of surveillance, censorship and repression, have been erected and implemented in many 'liberal democracies', including Australia, in the seventeen years since the launch of the infamous 'war on terror'. Geopolitical rivalries and anti-foreigner discourse and sentiment are ratcheting up. As Mariam Issa put it so well, a critical choice before us is to overcome fear, ignorance and intolerance through the acceptance of our inherent vulnerability that comes with a deeper understanding of our interdependence and interconnection – both amongst us as human beings and with the broader community of life on which we all depend in a myriad of ways (chapter 1). Farmers know this all too well: the soil is both the hero and the foundation of sustainable food systems, a truth emphasised by Graham and Annemarie Brookman, Liz Clay, Steve Hoepfner and Joel Orchard.

CONCLUSION

The urban farms described in these pages were, in many cases, established in places that were far from ideal and (as is the case of the vast majority of Australia) in soils that were less than optimal. Yet, it has been through vision, passion, know-how, commitment and sheer hard work that abandoned, unloved and difficult plots from Perth to Adelaide to Mildura to Keilor East to Brisbane have been brought to a state of flourishing abundance and productivity. To paraphrase a famous German philosopher born 200 years ago: 'People make their own history, but not in circumstances of their own choosing'.[12] The world that confronts us is not ideal, and our capacity for action is subject to many obstacles and constraints. It is up to us in so many cases to make the best of a bad (or, at times, not so bad) lot. Are we going to be active shapers of our own history and creative narrators of our own stories? Or are we going to be passive observers, spectators of the historical process as it is written and shaped by the currently dominant actors?

The answer given by every contributor to this collection is a resounding, 'Yes! We will write our own history!' These are individuals who have taken risks, who have made long and arduous physical, emotional and intellectual journeys, who have faced their fears and are living their dreams. Each story of urban farming narrated in this collection is a source of inspiration and wisdom, borne of years of experimentation, learning, reflection and action. We are inspired by micro-, home-based urban agriculture, in the form of Mariam Issa's R.A.W. garden in Brighton (chapter 1) and the garden farming of Kat Lavers in Northcote and Hannah Moloney in Hobart (chapter 5). We are excited about the community-level production underway in the pioneering Food Next Door collaboration between local community food activists and members of the Burundian community in Mildura (chapter 3) and about the equally inspiring, but also tragic, story of Urban Food Street in Buderim in the Sunshine Coast, wonderfully and thoughtfully told by Caroline Kemp (chapter 13). We delighted in Steve Hoepfner's account of the experimentation and collaboration amongst friends that led to the establishment of Wagtail Urban Farm in Adelaide (chapter 10) and in the cultural enrichment and, at times, life-saving properties of the dozens of allotment gardens facilitated across Melbourne by Cultivating Community, thanks to

Peta Christensen (chapter 4). Morag Gamble shared her passionate story (chapter 8) of a decades-long journey of community food systems and permaculture practice, from the very beginnings of Northey Street City Farm in Brisbane, one of a handful of rich cultural and highly productive assets created in a small number of Australian cities by grassroots community members.

We were privileged to share a number of stories of commercial-scale urban and peri-urban farming in different locations across Australia. We feasted with Gabriella Gomersall-Hubbard on the fabulous creation of a little piece of Calabria by Tony and Lina Siciliano at Rose Creek Estate in Keilor East (chapter 2). We rejoiced in the abundant yields of the permaculture Food Forest created in harsh conditions outside Adelaide by Graham and Annemarie Brookman (chapter 6), who learnt from their environment and experimented with techniques and species, adapting their farming practices to meet the challenges of their country. We celebrated Joel Orchard's journey to 'punk farming' (chapter 12) with the creation of Future Feeders in Mullumbimby and now the development of a Young Farmers Network for Australia. Toby Whittington and Ali Sumner's Perth-based social enterprise, Green World Revolution (chapter 9), has shown that it is possible for urban farming on small city blocks to be commercially viable and address some of the most difficult social problems at the same time – in this case, long-term unemployment and the social isolation and mental health issues that accompany it. Similarly, Vanessa Kwiatkowski and Mat Lumalasi have demonstrated that there is not only a future for urban rooftop and backyard honey in Australia, but hopefully also a future for the bees on which so much of our food system depends (chapter 11). Together, these are illustrative of the forms of urban commoning articulated by Katherine Gibson, which inspired the title and framing of the stories in this book.

As Katherine wrote in her introductory chapter, the commons is best understood as a process and set of practices, as much as, if not more than, a physical collection of resources and materials. It is in many ways a verb rather than a noun, hence the reference to *commoning*. *Commoning* describes a diverse and expanding array of practices and interactions that are expressive of new forms of social relations, between and amongst groups of people, and between people and other lifeforms. This is what we had in mind when we conceived of *Reclaiming the Urban Commons*. It was an invitation to our contributors both to share their individual stories of urban and peri-urban agriculture in all their diversity and particularity, as well as to reflect on what lessons they had learnt along the way that might provide inspiration and hope for the Australian community more broadly.

As we mentioned in the overview of this anthology, there are themes that resonate across the chapters that capture much of the essence of new forms of social relations that represent contemporary forms of urban food system commoning in Australia. These themes include:

- *sharing and collaboration* (of resources, of knowledge, of skills, of land, of traditions and culture, of food);
- *connection and interdependence* (to country, to place, to home, to history and memories, to friends and community);
- *nurturing, care, respect and trust* (of women, of children, of cultural difference, of multiple species, of life itself);
- *celebration, joy, welcoming and hospitality;*
- *healing and overcoming* (of divisions, of fear, of ignorance and bigotry, of past and present suffering and injustice);
- *creativity* (to imagine, to transform, to work with plants and animals, to co-design); and
- *diversity* (of plants, of species, of cultures, of people).

These are the values, principles and ways of living, working and being that speak to our higher potential, to our better selves. As Mariam Issa put it:

> *Both our individual and collective worlds are in transition and humanity is going through the remembrance of our true ideal: creating a sustainable world for each other.*

This is the aspiration shared by every contributor to this anthology and, we believe, very broadly across the Australian community and beyond. Remember, the stories shared in this anthology are but a small snapshot of a rapidly unfolding movement across Australia and globally. Governments in our country and worldwide have committed to this aspiration in the Sustainable Development Goals. How do we get from our current situation of unsustainability to a future in which all life can flourish?

The solutions are already all around us, as Graham and Annemarie Brookman said. They have been narrated in the stories in these pages; there is inspiration and support for all who want to join the new generation of commoners. If you are connected to a school, help it establish an edible garden. Join your local community garden or start one with your friends. Help your local council understand the value of edible urban landscapes and streetscapes; send your councillors the Urban Agriculture Manifesto in the appendix. Find ways to connect with local producers, if you haven't already.

The future, as Canadian author William Gibson observed many years ago, is already here. It's just not evenly distributed. Our job is to bring about a more even distribution, and in so doing, to both reclaim and usher in the age of the *Urban Commons*. Every time you plant a seed and care for the soil and the vast life within it, you are doing exactly that.

Appendix

The Urban Agriculture Manifesto

In the final session of the 2018 national Urban Agriculture Forum, participants workshopped the draft Urban Agriculture Manifesto that we circulated prior to the event.

We are extremely grateful to all participants who engaged so thoroughly and thoughtfully with this text. Below, we reproduce the revised text, which we hope has done justice to the discussions and edits made during the forum.

This document is intended to present a considered, coherent and visionary agenda for major change to support this sector's aspirations for a flourishing, healthy, resilient and regenerative food system. We believe it is achievable and necessary. While it is directed, in the first instance, towards the Victorian government, we believe it sets out an agenda for change that can be adapted and taken up nationally. We call on all our supporters and those who share the vision of a better food system to send this document to their MPs and political representatives.

The Urban Agriculture Forum Statement: Urban and Peri-Urban Agriculture Food System Renewal Manifesto

Revised at the second national Urban Agriculture Forum, 23–24 February 2018, William Angliss Institute, Melbourne

Introduction

We live in an era of systemic crisis. Daily, we see and hear stories attesting to the inherent unsustainability of the many systems that govern our lives. The most fundamentally important story, and the one that has the greatest impact, is the food system: everything that happens from soil to stomach that enables humanity to feed itself. By changing the food system, we can successfully meet the challenges of this century. Making cities edible by growing food in, around and near to them – urban and peri-urban agriculture – has a major role to play in supporting this necessary transformation. It is an idea for which the time has come.

The crisis is also manifest in social, physical and mental health impacts. Dietary-related disease is the biggest public health issue facing Australia. Our daily lives are relentlessly fast and busy, yet, increasingly, people report high levels of social isolation. More than ever before, we are disconnected from the social reality and ecology of our food system and from each other.

Acknowledging this disconnection, we have come together to discuss ways that these problems can be addressed through necessary and urgent changes to the current food system. We believe that a vital part of a positive new system is sustainable urban agriculture.

The Forum Statement

We, the attendees of the Sustain Urban Agriculture Forum, meeting on Wurundjeri Land, acknowledging Elders past, present and future, and recognising Indigenous wisdom and multi-generational stewardship of the land now called Australia, call on the Victorian State Government to acknowledge and support the renewal of the Victorian food system to:

1. Recognise the critical role that sustainable rural, regional, urban and peri-urban agriculture plays in achieving multi-generational food security, to be achieved through:
    1.1. Explicitly recognising urban agriculture as a permitted use in residential, commercial and mixed-use zones in the *Planning and Environment Act*;
    1.2. Creating and implementing a sustainable urban and peri-urban agriculture and land-use strategy, linked to multi-generational food security objectives;
    1.3. Comprehensively mapping and permanently protecting all remaining high-value farmland within 200 kilometres of the CBD, linking this to productive corridors radiating outwards to all regional centres;
    1.4. Creating dedicated urban and peri-urban agriculture zones within each of the existing twelve Green Wedge areas;
    1.5. Supporting dedicated urban farms and market gardens, and associated public produce markets, throughout our cities, towns and suburbs;
    1.6. Creating an urban agriculture fund to support community groups, not-for-profits and social enterprises; and
    1.7. Fostering intra- and inter-state collaboration with other local and state governments to promote a shared state-wide and national agenda for a healthy, sustainable and fair food system.

APPENDIX

2. Acknowledge that FOOD IS FUNDAMENTAL TO LIFE and that major changes to the food system are required to support Victorians' desire to enjoy a healthy and happy life, in connection with other people and nature, by:
    2.1. Acknowledging Indigenous food knowledge and traditions, integrating this into school curricula and supporting Victorian Aboriginal communities to cultivate their traditional grains and edible plants;
    2.2. Mandating that every Victorian school have an edible garden and incorporate food growing, cooking and nutrition into the school curriculum;
    2.3. Instigating food system literacy targets for all Victorian school children; and
    2.4. Supporting and expanding the handful of pilot programs connecting school children with farms.

3. Recognise that sustainable rural, regional, urban and peri-urban agriculture builds soil health, increases ecosystem resilience, encourages biodiversity and regenerates polluted waterways (Regenerative Food System), and therefore direct food and agriculture policy and programs to:
    3.1. Protect our soils, waterways and ecosystems;
    3.2. Work closely with Indigenous elders in all places, acknowledging and respecting Indigenous food sovereignty and land management;
    3.3. Recognise and celebrate the leadership that many farmers at all scales and in all places (rural, regional and urban/peri-urban) are providing to help us transition to a Regenerative Food System;
    3.4. Support market gardeners and farmers to transition to sustainable and regenerative forms of horticulture and agriculture;
    3.5. Renew efforts to connect people with the source of their food; and
    3.6. Serve the interests of all life, now and in the future.

4. Protect the health and wellbeing of Victorians, especially the most vulnerable, by:
   4.1. Amending the *Planning and Environment Act* to make assessments of the health, wellbeing and environmental impacts of fast food retail outlets mandatory in planning approvals;[1]
   4.2. Prohibiting the opening of new fast-food outlets within 1 kilometre of educational and/or healthcare facilities, and reducing the density of existing fast-food outlets near educational and healthcare facilities, recognising the vulnerability of lower socioeconomic areas to this industry; and
   4.3. Advocating for strict controls on the advertising of fast foods and sugary sweetened beverages to audiences that include children and youth under eighteen.

5. Understand that FOOD IS BASIC TO HUMAN AND ECOSYSTEM PROSPERITY AND FLOURISHING in diverse monetary and non-monetary ways.

6. Recognise that FOOD IS CENTRAL TO CULTURAL VITALITY and value the importance of a food system in which all people know where their food comes from, appreciate different food cultures and learn how to eat well so they can enjoy healthy food every day.

7. Recognise that FOOD IS DEEPLY POLITICAL, that it affects us all and, therefore, we must all have a voice in its current and future direction.

Notes

Overview
1. T. Berry, *The Great Work: Our Way into the Future*, Crown, 2000.

Introduction: Food as Urban Commons and Community Economics
1. S. Gudeman, *The Anthropology of Economy: Commodity, Market, and Culture*, Blackwell Publishers, Oxford, 2001, p. 27.
2. A. Huron, *Carving out the Commons: Tenant Organizing and Housing Cooperatives in Washington D.C.*, University of Minnesota Press, Minneapolis, 2018, p. 64.
3. P. Linebaugh, *The Magna Carta Manifesto: Liberties and Commons for All*, University of California Press, Berkley, 2018.
4. J. K. Gibson-Graham, J. Cameron & S. Healy, *Take Back the Economy: An Ethical Guide for Transforming Our Communities*, University of Minnesota Press, Minneapolis, 2013.
5. W. Steffen, W. Broadgate, L. Deutsch, O. Gaffney & C. Ludwig, 'The trajectory of the Anthropocene: The Great Acceleration', *The Anthropocene Review*, vol. 2, no. 1, 2015, pp. 81–98.
6. R. Grayson, 'An Interview about Footpath Gardens Raises Questions', *Australian City Farms and Community Gardens Network Newsletter*, April 2017, viewed 16 July 2018, <https://communitygarden.org.au/an-interview-about-footpath-gardens-raises-questions/>.
7. J. Cameron, *The Newcastle Community Garden Project*, Placestories, 2010, viewed 6 June 2018, <http://placestories.com/ project/7733>.
8. R. Powell, 'Gardening: A DIY Gardening Project Helps Migrants and Refugees at Mamre House', *Sydney Morning Herald*, 5 February 2017, viewed 6 June 2018, <https://www.smh.com.au/entertainment/gardening-a-diy-garden-project-helps-migrants-and-refugees-at-mamre-house-20160204-gmlpcp.html>.
9. J. K. Gibson-Graham, J. Cameron & S. Healy, *Take Back the Economy: An Ethical Guide for Transforming Our Communities*, University of Minnesota Press, Minnesota, 2013.

NOTES

Chapter 2 – Preserving Calabrian Traditions in the Suburbs: Rose Creek Estate, East Keilor

1. More detailed information on Rose Creek Estate can be found in G. Gomersall-Hubbard, *Growing Honest Food – An Oasis of Italian Tradition in the Suburbs*, Hyland House Publishing, Melbourne, 2012.
2. Rose Creek Estate, <www.rosecreekestate.com.au>.
3. Tony and Lina take their produce to the Slow Food (Abbotsord Convent), Gasworks (Albert Park) and Collingwood Children's Farm markets. For more information, see Victorian Farmer's Markets Association, <www.vfma.org.au>.
4. For example, Melbourne Food and Wine Festival Events: The Crushed Olive, Rose Creek Estate 2 April 2017; and A Toast to Vendemmia (grape harvest), Rose Creek Estate, 18 March 2018.
5. For example, Diggers Club, Traditional Italian Regional Cooking Masterclass, Garden of St. Erth, Blackwood, 16 November 2014; Diggers Club, Melbourne International Flower and Garden Show, Cooking with Heirloom Tomatoes.
6. R. Foskey, *Older Farmers and Retirement: A Report for the Rural Industries Research and Development Corporation (RIRDC)*, Australian Government, RIRDC, Canberra, 2005, viewed 6 June 2018, <http://www.agrifutures.com.au/wp-content/uploads/publications/05-006.pdf>.
7. National Centre for Farmer Health, *Farm Succession Planning*, viewed 20 March 2017, <www.farmerhealth.org.au/page/health-centre/farm-succession-planning>; N. Shady & A. Hilton, *Who Gets the Farm? A Practical Guide to Farm Succession*, Global Publishing Group, February 2006.
8. Foskey, *Older Farmers and Retirement*.
9. A. Marshall, 'Transitions Options Help Older Farmers and New Work Together', *The Land*, 3 August 2016, <www.theland.com.au>. Intervale Centre, a non profit organisation in Burlington, Vermont, USA, runs 325 acres of reclaimed agricultural land. It is a model for food and farming organisations, promoting food systems that support communities, sustainable use of land and farm incubators <www.intervale.org>.

Chapter 3 – Bringing Together Landless Farmers and Unused Farmland: The Sunraysia Burundian Garden and Food Next Door Initiative

1. Australian Bureau of Statistics (ABS), *Mildura Local Government Area (LGA), 2016 Census QuickStats*, ABS, Canberra, 2017, viewed 13 October 2017, <www.censusdata.abs.gov.au/census_services/getproduct/census/2016/quickstat/LGA24780?opendocument>; ABS, *Robinvale Statistical Area Level 2, 2016 Census QuickStats*, ABS, Canberra, 2017, viewed 13 October 2017, <www.censusdata.abs.gov.au/census_services/getproduct/census/2016/quickstat/215031403?opendocument>; ABS, *Wentworth Local Government Area (LGA), 2016 Census QuickStats*, ABS, Canberra, 2017, viewed 13 October 2017, <www.censusdata.abs.gov.au/census_services/getproduct/census/2016/quickstat/LGA18200?opendocument>.
2. Traditional Aboriginal custodians of the area are the Latji Latji, Paakantji (Barkindji), Ngiyampaa, Mutthi Mutthi, Wemba Wemba and Tati Tati and Barapa Barapa; Mallee District Aboriginal Services (MDAS), *Cultural History*, MDAS, Mildura, 2013, viewed 13 October 2017, <www.mdas.org.au/ABOUT-MDAS/Cultural-History.aspx>.

NOTES

3   J. A. La Nauze, *Alfred Deakin: A Biography*, Melbourne University Press, Carlton, 1965; B. Rankin, 'Alfred Deakin and Water Resources Politics in Australia', *History Australia*, vol. 10. no. 2. 2013, pp. 114–35.
4   Mildura Development Corporation (MDC), *2014 Regional Overview Mildura-Wentworth*, MDC, Mildura, 2014.
5   ibid; T, Spaven, 'Exploring Migrants' Contributions to Agriculture: The Story of Italians in the Sunraysia Region', unpublished honours thesis, University of Wollongong, NSW, 2016.
6   Mildura Rural City Council (MRCC), *VLGA Food Scan Report: Mildura Rural City Council*, MRCC, Mildura, 2013; Victorian Department of Economic Development, Jobs, Transport and Resources (DEDJTR), *Fruit and Nut Industries Profile*, DEDJTR, Melbourne, 2014, viewed 16 March 2018, <http://agriculture.vic.gov.au/agriculture/horticulture>; DEDJTR, *Grape Industries Profile*, Melbourne, 2014, viewed 16 March 2018, <http://agriculture.vic.gov.au/agriculture/horticulture>.
7   B. Missingham, J. Dibden, & C. Cocklin, 'A Multicultural Countryside? Ethnic Minorities in Rural Australia', *Rural Society*, vol. 16, no. 2, 2006, pp. 131–50.
8   Instigated by the Refugee Council of Australia, 'a Refugee Welcome Zone is a is a Local Government Area which has made a commitment in spirit to welcoming refugees into the community, upholding the human rights of refugees, demonstrating compassion for refugees and enhancing cultural and religious diversity in the community'; Mildura Rural City Council (MRCC), *Refugee Welcome Zone*, MRCC, Mildura, 2017, viewed 13 October 2017, <www.mildura.vic.gov.au/Community/Refugee-Welcome-Zone>.
9   MRCC, *VLGA Food Scan Report: Mildura Rural City Council*, MRCC, Mildura, 2013, p. 29, viewed 13 October 2017, <www.healthytogethermildura.com.au/wp-content/uploads/2013/06/061013_VLGA_Scan_Report_HTMildura_Report_V1.3.pdf>.
10 ibid.
11 Key factors were changing economic structures (associated with agricultural imports and deregulation of the dried fruit industry), low commodity prices (especially for wine grapes), a new deregulated water system (characterised by decreased water allocations, unbundled land and water rights, and tradeable water), implementation of the Murray Darling Basin plan, and intergenerational succession issues on family farms; Mallee Catchment Management Authority (Mallee CMA), *Drought Impact 2008–09: Irrigation Status Report for the Sunraysia Pumped Irrigation Districts*, Mallee CMA, Mildura, 2009, viewed 2 November 2016, <www.malleecma.vic.gov.au/resources/fact-sheets/irrigationstatusreport_final.pdf>; L. Head, M. Adams, H. V. McGregor & S. Toole, 'Climate Change and Australia', *Wiley Interdisciplinary Reviews: Climate Change*, vol. 5, no. 2, 2014, pp. 175–197; L. Head, N. Klocker, O. Dun & T. Spaven, 'Irrigator Relations with Water in the Sunraysia Region, Northwestern Victoria', *Geographical Research*, vol. 56, no. 1, 2018, pp. 92–106; A. S. Kiem & E. K. Austin, 'Drought and the Future of Rural Communities: Opportunities and Challenges for Climate Change Adaptation in Regional Victoria, Australia', *Global Environmental Change*, vol. 23, no. 5, 2013, pp. 1307–16; T. Spaven, 'Exploring Migrants' Contributions to Agriculture: The Story of Italians in the Sunraysia Region', Honours dissertation, University of Wollongong, 2016.
12 A. S. Kiem, L. E. Askew, M. Sherval, D.C. Verdon-Kidd, C. Clifton, E. Austin, P. M. McGuirk, & H. Berry, *Drought and the Future of Rural Communities:*

NOTES

Drought Impacts and Adaptation in Regional Victoria, National Climate Change Adaptation Research Facility, Gold Coast, 2010, viewed 6 June 2018, <www.nccarf.edu.au/sites/default/files/attached_files_publications/Kiem_2010_Drought_and_small_inland_settlements.pdf>.

13   Unpublished notes from Mildura Development Corporation (MDC), 2016 about the multi-agency Sunraysia Rejuvenation Project, which was tasked with bringing 'the dried off areas in existing irrigation districts back into agricultural production (rejuvenation); Lower Murray Water (LMW), *2018–2023 Price Submission – Rural*, 28 September 2017, LMW, Mildura, p. 19, viewed 19 February 2018, <www.esc.vic.gov.au/sites/default/files/documents/2018-water-price-review-lower-murray-water-price-submission-rural-20170928.pdf>.

14   This research was conducted under an Australian Research Council grant (DP140101165 - 'Sustainability and climate change adaptation: Unlocking the potential of ethnic diversity') awarded to Lesley Head, Natascha Klocker, Gordon Waitt and Heather Goodall in 2014.

15   Mildura Rural City Council (MRCC), *New and Emerging Communities Plan*, MRCC, Mildura, 2015, viewed 6 June 2018, <www.mildura.vic.gov.au/Community/Community-Plans>.

16   Sunraysia Mallee Ethnic Communities Council (SMECC), *Food Next Door – Burundian garden project*, SMECC, Mildura, 2016, viewed 13 October 2017, <www.smeccinc.org/food-next-door---burundian-garden-project.html>.

17   E. Brown, 'Out of Africa: The Community Project Involving Food and Farming Bringing New Migrants Together', *Australian Broadcasting Corporation (ABC)*, Sydney, 2017, viewed 6 June 2018 <www.abc.net.au/tv/programs/landline/old-site/content/2017/s4650651.htm>; M. Frankel-Vaughan, 'Burundian Garden Opening: Food Project A-maize-ing,' *Sunraysia Daily*, 24 September 2016, viewed 6 June 2018, <www.sunraysiadaily.com.au/story/4185995/burundian-garden-opening-food-project-a-maize-ing/>; D. White, 'Growing Together,' *Sunraysia Daily*, 19 February 2017, viewed 6 June 2018, <www.sunraysiadaily.com.au/story/4477783/growing-together/>.

18   An alternative food system that enhances access to fresh fruit and vegetables; reduces environmental impacts; improves food security for low income, disadvantaged and marginalised groups; and connects people eating food to those growing it; Urban Agriculture Forum, *What is Urban Agriculture?*, Sustain, Melbourne, n.d., viewed 19 February 2018, <www.uaf.org.au/about-urban-agriculture>.

19   Facebook, viewed 17 July 2018, <www.facebook.com/foodnextdoorcoop/>.

Chapter 4 – Cultivating Community

1   Cultivating Community, Richmond, 2018, viewed 6 June 2018, <www.cultivatingcommunity.org.au>.

Chapter 5 – Unearthing the Potential of Home Food Production

1   SBS Australia, *Community Environment Park's Food Miles Report*, Sydney, 2018, viewed 6 June 2018, <www.sbs.com.au/shows/foodinvestigators/listings/detail/i/1/article/2941/Food-Miles>.

2   P. Wise, *Grow Your Own: The Potential Value and Impacts of Residential and Community Food Gardening*, The Australia Institute, Canberra, p. 59, viewed 6 June 2018, <www.tai.org.au/sites/defualt/files/PB%2059%20Grow%20Your%20Own.pdf>.

NOTES

3   C. Blazey & J. Varkulevicius, *The Australian Fruit and Vegetable Garden: Grow the Best Fruit and Vegetable for Good Health and Flavour*, Diggers Club, Vic, 2006.

4   Affordable testing for home gardeners is available through Macquarie University's *VegeSafe* program. Macquarie University, *VegeSafe*, Sydney, 2018, viewed 6 June 2018, <https://research.science.mq.edu.au/vegesafe/>.

5   The Lead Group, *Lead Action News*, NSW, 2018, viewed 6 June 2018, <www.lead.org.au/fs/fst6.html>; C. J. Rosen, *Lead in the Home Garden and Urban Soil Environment*, University of Minnesota, MN, 2018, viewed 6 June 2018 <www.extension.umn.edu/garden/yard-garden/soils/lead-in-home-garden/>.

6   It's important to note that while permaculture thinking can also be applied to building, transportation, technology, economics, education, governance and health and wellbeing, in this chapter we'll focus on our lived experience of land management at the suburban, household scale. D. Holmgren, *About Permaculture*, Holmgren Design, Vic., 2018, viewed 6 June 2018, <www.holmgren.com.au/about-permaculture/>.

7   D. Holmgren, *RetroSuburbia: A Downshifter's Guide to a Resilient Future*, Melliodora Publishing, Vic., 2018.

8   The Willing Workers on Organic Farms (WWOOF) network connects growers (including urban growers) with volunteers to swap food, accommodation and hands-on learning for a helping hand, and has been an invaluable immersive learning experience for many in the urban agriculture movement.

Chapter 7 – Garden Farming: The Foundation for Agriculturally Productive Cities and Towns

1   D. Holmgren, *RetroSuburbia: The Downshifter's Guide to a Resilient Future*, Melliodara Publishing, Vic., 2018.

2   Greywater is household wastewater from bathrooms, laundries and kitchens without human faecal contamination.

3   'Humanure' is a term coined by Joseph Jenkins to recognise human waste as just another organic fertiliser.

4   D. Holmgren, *Feeding Retrosuburbia: From the Backyard to the Bioregion*, viewed June 6 2018 < www.retrosuburbia.com/wp-content/uploads/2017/10/Feeding_RetroSuburbia_eBook.pdf>.

5   The Bank for International Settlements says Australia's fifty-five-year house price 'upswing' is the longest in the world; G. D. Sutton, D. Mihaljek & A. Subelyte, *Interest Rates and House Prices in the United States and Around the World*, Bank for International Settlements (BIS), Switzerland, 2017, viewed 6 June 2018, <www.bis.org/publ/work665.pdf>.

6   R. Hopkins, *The Transition Handbook: Creating Local Sustainable Communities Beyond Oil Dependency*, Finch Publishing, NSW, 2009.

7   Permablitz, *About Permablitz*, Melbourne, 2018, viewed 6 June 2018, <www.permablitz.net/about-permablitz>.

8   D. Holmgren, *RetroSuburbia: The Downshifter's Guide to a Resilient Future*, pp. 67, 234–7.

9   The Australian Industry Group (AIG), *A Supply Chain Based Approach to Carbon Abatement: Pilot Study*, AIG, Sydney 2011.

10   Holmgren, *Feeding Retrosuburbia*.

11   R. Hopkins, *Ingredients of Transition: The Great Reskilling*, Transition Culture, Devon, 2010, viewed 9 May 2018, <https://www.transitionculture.org/2010/10/05/ingredients-of-transition-the-great-reskilling/>.

12   D. Holmgren, *Future Scenarios: How Communities Can Adapt to Peak Oil and Climate Change*, Chelsea Green, White River Junction, VT, 2009.

13   Increasing immigration might be one unpopular option that may increase social friction.

14   J. Daley, B. Coates & T. Wiltshire, *Housing Affordability: Re-imagining the Australian Dream: Grattan Institute Report No. 2018-04*, Grattan Institute, VIC, 2018, viewed 6 June 2018; P. Newman, T. Beatley & H. Boyer, *Resilient Cities Second Edition: Overcoming Fossil Fuel Dependence*, Island Press, Washington, DC.

15   In 'Retrofitting the Suburbs for Sustainability', I show how policies, affluence and other factors driving more construction in our residential streets lead to a decrease rather than an increase in population density; D. Holmgren, *Retrofitting the Suburbs for the Energy Descent Future: Simplicity Institute Report 12i*, Simplicity Institute, VIC, 2012, viewed 6 June 2018, <https://holmgren.com.au/wp-content/uploads/2003/11/RetrofittingTheSuburbsSimplicityInstitute1.pdf>.

16   H. Pawson, Taxing Empty Homes: A Step Towards Affordable Housing, but Much More can be Done, *The Conversation*, 17 July 2017, viewed 9 May 2018, <https://theconversation.com/taxing-empty-homes-a-step-towards-affordable-housing-but-much-more-can-be-done-80742>.

17   A. Mitchelson, Loneliness is a condition that rivals smoking, obesity, *The New Daily*, 7 August 2017, viewed 6 June 2018, <https://thenewdaily.com.au/life/wellbeing/2017/08/07/loneliness-epidemic-obesity-isolation/>.

Chapter 8 – Citizen Design, Permaculture and Community-based Urban Agriculture

1   E. Resnick, *Developing Citizen Designers*, Bloomsbury Academic, Sydney, 2016.

2   J. Chisholm, *What is Co-design*, Design For Europe, United Kingdom, 2018, viewed 6 June 2018, <http://designforeurope.eu/what-co-design>.

3   Citizen Designer, *Everyday People Making the City*, 2018, viewed 6 June 2018, <http://www.citizendesigner.org>.

4   Transition Network, United Kingdom, 2016, viewed 6 June 2018, <http://transitionnetwork.org/>.

Chapter 9 – Green World Revolution: Urban Farming as Social Enterprise

1   T. Barone, 'Crime Pockets point to historic social problems,' *The West Australian*, Saturday 17 August 2013, viewed 6 June 2018, <https://thewest.com.au/news/wa/crime-pockets-point-to-historic-social-problems-ng-ya-355781>.

2   Social Policy Research Centre (SPRC), *Poverty in Australia 2016: Poverty and Inequality in Australia Series* (5th Ed.), Australian Council of Social Services, NSW, 2016, viewed 6 June 2018, <www.acoss.org.au/wp-content/uploads/2016/10/Poverty-in-Australia-2016.pdf>.

3   Social Traders, *What is Social Enterprise. Social Enterprise Definition*, Social Traders, Melbourne, 2018, viewed 10 March 2018, <www.socialtraders.com.au/about-social-enterprise/what-is-a-social-enterprise/social-enterprise-definition/>.

4   D. Kolb, *Experiential Learning: Experience as the Source of Learning and Development*, (2nd ed.), Pearson Education, New Jersey, 2015.

5   W. K. Kellogg Foundation, *Logic Model Development Guide*, Kellogg Foundation, Michigan, 2006, viewed 6 June 2018 <https://www.wkkf.org/resource-directory/resource/2006/02/wk-kellogg-foundation-logic-model-development-guide>.

6   E. de Bono, *Six Thinking Hats*, Viking, United Kingdom, 1986; E. de Bono, *The Power of Perception. Ten Thinking Tools for Making Better Business Decisions*,

NOTES

de Bono Thinking Systems, USA, 2009; E. de Bono, *Lateral Thinking. Fast Track to Creativity*, de Bono Thinking Systems, USA, 2009.

Chapter 11 – Melbourne City Rooftop Honey

1. Rural Industries Research and Development Corporation (RIRDC), *The Real Value of Pollination*, Pollination Fact Sheet, Australian Government, RIRDC, Canberra, 2010, viewed 6 June 2018, <https://honeybee.org.au/pdf/PollinationAwareFactSheet.pdf>.
2. L. Johnson, *City Farmer: Adventures in Urban Food Growing*, Greystone Books Ltd, USA, 2011; P. Ladner, *The Urban Food Revolution: Changing the Way We Feed Cities*, New Society Publishers, Canada, 2011; articles by C. Blazey in *The Diggers Club Magazine*; J. Cockrall-King, *Food and the City: Urban Agriculture and the New Food Revolution*, Prometheus Books, NY, 2012; R. Shulman, *Eat the City: A Tale of the Fishers, Foragers, Butchers, Farmers, Poultry Minders*, Crown Archetype, MA, 2013; R. Anderson, *Whole Larder Love: Grow, Gather, Hunt, Cook*, Penguin Books Australia, Melbourne, 2012.
3. H. Schofield, 'Paris Fast Becoming Queen Bee of the Urban Apiary World', BBC News Europe, 14 August 2010, viewed 6 June 2018, <www.bbc.co.uk/news/world-europe-10942618>.

Chapter 12 – Farming is Punk

1. M. Fukouka, *The One-straw Revolution: An Introduction to Natural Farming*, New York Review of Books, NY, 2010.

Chapter 13 – Urban Food Street

1. Australian term for a piece of publicly owned land between the front boundary of a house or other building and the street, typically grassed and maintained either by the house owner or local authority, but often by neither.
2. 'Food miles' is part of the broader issue of sustainability that deals with a wide range of economic, environmental and social issues, including 'local food'. The term 'food miles' was coined by Professor Tim Lang (Food Policy, City University London), who notes: 'The point was to highlight the hidden ecological, social and economic consequences of food production to consumers in a simple way, one which had objective reality but also connotations'; T. Lang & M. Heasman, *Food Wars: The Global Battle for Mouths, Minds and Markets* (2nd ed.), Routledge, London, pp. 94–97; T. Lang, *Locale/Globale (Food Miles)*, Slow Food, Italy, 2006, viewed 6 June 2018, <www.city.ac.uk/__data/assets/pdf_file/0007/167893/Slow-Food-fd-miles-final-16-02-06.pdf>.
3. Project for Public Spaces (PPS) is a non-profit organisation dedicated to helping people create and sustain public spaces that build strong communities. It is the central hub of the global placemaking movement and connects people to ideas, resources, expertise and partners who see *place* as the key to addressing our greatest challenges.
4. Urban Food Street, Qld., 2017, viewed 6 June 2018, <www.urbanfoodstreet.com>.
5. J. Risom & M. Madriz, *Embracing the Paradox of Planning for Informality*, Next City, PA, 1 January 2018, viewed 6 June 2018, <http://nextcity.org/features/view/embracing-the-paradox-of-planning-for-informality>.
6. Design-thinking utilises elements from the designer's toolkit, such as empathy and experimentation, to arrive at innovative solutions. By using design-thinking,

a decision is made based on the consideration of users' real, current and future needs, instead of relying on empirical data or evidence-less 'hunches'.

7   'Ageing in place' is a 'term used to describe a person living in the residence of their choice, for as long as they are able, as they age. This includes being able to have any services (or other support) they might need over time as their needs change'; Age in Place (AiP), *What is Aging in Place*, AiP, TN, 2018, viewed 6 June 2018 <https://ageinplace.com/aging-in-place-basics/what-is-aging-in-place/>.

8   Published in 2010 by print publication Architecture AU as an edited version of Ken Maher's 2009 AS Hook Address. We adopted this quote and used it on noticeboards around the neighbourhood to advise the public of the ethos that was guiding the project; ArchitectureAu (AAu), *An Architecture of Engagement: The 2009 A. S. Hook Address by Gold Medallist Ken Maher*, Architecture Media Pty ltd, VIC, 2018, viewed 6 June 2018, <https://architectureau.com/articles/an-architecture-of-engagement/>.

9   R. Boyd, *The Australian Ugliness*, Cheshire, Melbourne, 1960..

10 Z. Myers, Street Eats: From Suburban Wasteland to Community Kitchen, *Foreground*, Australia, 19 September 2017, viewed 6 June 2018, <www.foreground.com.au/public-domain/suburban-wasteland-community-kitchen>.

11 Jane Jacobs, in *The Death and Life of Great American Cities* identifies the three main qualities that 'a city street equipped to handle strangers, and to make a safety asset, in itself, of the presence of strangers' must have, namely a clear demarcation between public and private spaces, buildings oriented to the street, and continuous pedestrian use of sidewalks in order to maintain eyes on the street'; J. Jacobs, *The Death and Life of Great American Cities*, Random House, NY, 2002 (1961), p. 35.

12 This is one of the key attributes of the Swedish concept of co-housing: an intentional community of private homes clustered around shared outdoor space, which may include parking, walkways, open space and gardens. Households have independent incomes and private lives, but neighbours collaboratively plan and manage community activities and shared spaces. Co-housing makes it easy to carpool, form clubs, share resources such as tools and cars, and organise child and elder care.

Chapter 14 – Learning From our Productive Past

1   G. Pickering (ed.), *Fanny Balbuk Yoreel, Realising a Perth Resistance Fighter*, National Trust of Western Australia, Perth, 2017, viwed 6 June 2018, <https://www.nationaltrust.org.au/publications/fanny-balbuk-perth-resistance-fighter/>; Western Australiam Museum, *Reimagining Perth's Lost Wetlands: Fanny Balbuk*, Government of Western Australia, Perth, 2018, viewed 6 June 2018, <http://museum.wa.gov.au/explore/wetlands/aboriginal-context/fanny-balbuk>.

2   Parliament of Victoria, Census of Victoria 1891, Part VII Land and Live Stock, Paper no. 34, *Votes and Proceedings of the Parliament of Victoria*, 1892–3, vol. 3. Government of Victoria, VIC.

3   A. Gaynor, 'Animal Agendas: Conflict Over Productive Animals in Twentieth-Century Australian Cities', *Society and Animals*, vol. 15, no. 1, 2007, pp. 29–42.

4   The productive features of historical Australian suburbia identified in this and subsequent paragraphs are discussed at length in A. Gaynor, *Harvest of the Suburbs: An Environmental History of Growing Food in Australian Cities*, UWA Press, Crawley, 2006, now available in creative commons licensed electronic format at www.environmentandsociety.org/node/8356.

NOTES

Chapter 15 – Feeding Melbourne: Market Gardening in the Sandbelt: 1950s–1970s
1   The Dingley bypass road never eventuated.

Chapter 16 – Australia, 1945: The Future Begins
1   P. Neruda, *Elemental Odes*, M. Sayers. Peden (trans), Libris, London, 1991.
2   A. Caldwell, *Commonwealth Parliamentary Debate – Arthur Calwell, August 1945*, Parliament of Australia, 2 August 1945, viewed 6 June 2018, <www.multiculturalaustralia.edu.au/doc/calwell_4.pdf>.
3   R. White, *Inventing Australia: Images and Identity, 1688–1980*, Allen & Unwin, Sydney, 1981, p. 71.
4   G. Megalogenis, *Australia's Second Chance, What our History Tells Us About Our Future*, Penguin Group Australia, Melbourne, 2015, p. 277.
5   B. Anderson, *Imagined Communities: Reflections on the Origin and Spread of Nationalism*, Verso, London, 1983.
6   S. Kunek, *Wives, Brides and Single Women: Greek female migration to Australia in the post-World War II period, 1945 to 1973*, PhD thesis, Monash University, VIC, 1994, chapters 3–5.
7   S. Kunek, *Wives, Brides and Single Women*, chapter 1.
8   S. McIntyre, *Australia's Boldest Experiment, War and Reconstruction in the 1940s*, NewSouth, NSW, 2015, pp. 333, 339.
9   G. Megalogenis, *Australia's Second Chance*, pp. 223, 241.
10   ibid., p. 251.
11   National Archives of Australia, *Australia's Prime Ministers: Harold Holt*, Australian Government, Canberra, 2016, viewed 7 March 2018, <http://primeministers.naa.gov.au/primeministers/holt/>.
12   Department of Home Affairs, *Fact Sheet – Abolition of the 'White Australia' Policy*, 2018, viewed 7 March 2018, <www.homeaffairs.gov.au/about/corporate/information/fact-sheets/08abolition>.
13   Foodbank (FB), *Foodbank Hunger Report 2017: Fighting Hunger in Australia* (FB), NSW, 2017, p. 6, viewed 6 June 2018, <www.foodbank.org.au/wp-content/uploads/2017/10/Foodbank-Hunger-Report-2017.pdf>.
14   S. McIntyre, *Australia's Boldest Experiment*, p. 88.
15   ibid., p. 1.
16   ibid., chapters 2–5.
17   S. McIntyre, *Australia's Boldest Experiment*, p. 343.
18   J. M. Keynes, *The General Theory of Employment, Interest and Money*, Palgrave Macmillan, London, 1936.
19   S. McIntyre, *Australia's Boldest Experiment*, pp. 87–8.
20   P. D. Phillips, F. W. Eggleston & K. H. Bailey, *The Peopling of Australia*, Melbourne University Press, Melbourne, 1933.
21   National Population Inquiry, W. D. Borrie & Department of Labor and Immigration, *Population and Australia, a Demographic Analysis and Projection: First Report of the National Population Inquiry*, vol. 1, Australian Government, Canberra, 1975, p. 193.
22   S. Kunek, *Wives, Brides and Single Women*, chapter 1.
23   Australia, House of Representatives, Debates, *Hansard*, vol. 184 (2 August 1945), 4911; R. L. Smith, 'Australian Immigration 1945–1974' in P. J. Brain, R. L. Smith & G. P. Schuyers, *Population, Immigration and the Australian Economy*, Croom Helm, London, 1979, pp. 59–73.

NOTES

24 S. Kunek, *Wives, Brides and Single Women*, chapters 3 and 5.
25 W. A. Sinclair, *The Process of Economic Development in Australia*, Cheshire, Melbourne, 1976, p. 235.
26 S. Kunek, *Wives, Brides and Single Women*, chapters 1–6.
27 S. McIntyre, *Australia's Boldest Experiment*, p. 363.
28 J. G. Crawford, *Wartime Agriculture in Australia and New Zealand 1939–50*, Stanford University Press, California, 1954.
29 Sir S. Wadham, R. K. Wilson & J. Wood, *Land Utilization in Australia*, Melbourne University Press, Melbourne, 1964, p. 263.
30 G. Megalogenis, *Australia's Second Chance*, p. 224.
31 ibid., p. 223.
32 V. Duma & H. Lichtenberger, 'Remembering Red Vienna', *Jacobin*, 2017, available at <www.jacobinmag.com/2017/02/red-vienna-austria-housing-urban-planning>.
33 S. McIntyre, *Australia's Boldest Experiment*, p. 409.
34 G. Megalogenis, *Australia's Second Chance*, pp. 235, 240–1.
35 ibid., p. 241.
36 ibid., p. 235.
37 C. Price, *Southern European Settlers in Australia*, Australian National University, Canberra, 1963, pp. 28, 30.
38 A. Abrams, *Why 'Urban Villages' are on the Rise Around the World*, Shareable, 2017, viewed 7 March 2018, <www.shareable.net/blog/why-urban-villages-are-on-the-rise-around-the-world>.
39 S. Kunek, *Navigating the Victorian Ethnic Food Trail* installation catalogue, Kunexion, Melbourne, 1996.
40 R. Broome, *The Victorians, Arriving*, Fairfax, Syme and Weldon Associated, Melbourne, 1984, p. 102–3.
41 J. Jupp, 'Australian Immigration 1788–1973', in F. Milne and P. Shergold (eds.), *The Great Immigration Debate*, Federation of Ethnic Communities Council of Australia, Sydney, 1984, p. 4.
42 R. Broome, *The Victorians*, pp. 112–15.
43 ibid., pp. 201–2.
44 C. Price, *Southern Europeans*, p. 3.
45 A. Mencke & T. van der Schafer, 'The Distribution of Dutch Immigrants in Australia', PhD thesis, School of Geography, University of Sydney, 1979, pp. 53, 57.
46 S. Kunek, Wives, *Brides and Single Women*, chapters 1–6.
47 ibid., chapter 6.
48 S. McIntyre, *Australia's Boldest Experiment*, pp. 87–9.
49 G. Megalogenis, *Australia's Second Chance*, pp. 247, 252, 257.
50 ibid., pp. 247–63, 267.
51 R. Millar & B. Schneiders, '4 Million, 5 Million, 8 Million: How Big is too Big for Liveable Melbourne?', *Age*, 3 July 2017, viewed 6 June 2018 <https://www.theage.com.au/national/victoria/4-million-5-million-8-million-how-big-is-too-big-for-liveable- melbourne-20170630-gx1u09.html>.
52 ibid.
53 T. Carr, K. Fernandez & T. Rosewall, 'The Recent Economic Performance of the States', *Bulletin*, March Quarter, 2017, pp. 3–4, viewed 6 June 2018, <www.rba.gov.au/publications/bulletin/2017/mar/1.html>.
54 Victorian Eco Innovation Lab (VEIL), *Melbourne's Food Future: Planning A Resilient City Food Bowl, A Foodprint Melbourne Report*, VEIL, Melbourne, 2016, p. 3, viewed 6 June 2018, <https://veil.msd.unimelb.edu.au/__data/assets/pdf_

NOTES

file/0008/2355146/Melbourne-Food-Future-planning-a-resilient-city-food-bowl-web.pdf>; VEIL, *Melbourne's Foodbowl, Now and at Seven Million, A Foodprint Melbourne Report*, VEIL, Melbourne, 2015, viewed 6 June 2018, <https://research.unimelb.edu.au/__data/assets/pdf_file/0008/2355155/Melbournes-Foodbowl-Now-and-at-seven-million.pdf>.

55 R. Millar & B. Schneiders, '4 million, 5 million, 8 million'.
56 J. Daley & B. Coates, *Housing Affordability Re-imagining the Australian Dream: Grattan Institute Report No. 2018-04*, Grattan Institute, VIC, March, 2018, viewed 6 June 2018, <https://grattan.edu.au/wp-content/uploads/2018/03/901-Housing-affordability.pdf>.

Conclusion – Laying the foundations for sustainable urban food systems in Australia

1 IPES-Food, *Too Big to Feed: Exploring the Impacts of Mega-mergers, Consolidation and, Concentration of Power in the Agri-food Sector*, 2017, <www.ipes-food.org/concentration>.
2 E. Holt-Gimenez, *A Foodie's Guide to Capitalism: Understanding the Political Economy of What We Eat*, NYU Press, New York, 2017.
3 G. Meyer, 'Cargill Profits Boosted by Growing Global Appetite for Meat', *Financial Times*, 13 July 2017, <www.ft.com/content/c4c0c184-5ce5-312f-b944-641d6675ba14>.
4 J. Hickel, 'The True Extent of Global Poverty and Hunger: Questioning the Good News Narrative of the Millennium Development Goals', *Third World Quarterly*, 2016, vol. 37, no. 5, pp. 1–19.
5 IPES-Food, 'Unravelling the Food–Health Nexus: Addressing Practices, Political Economy, and Power Relations to Build Healthier Food Systems', Global Alliance for the Future of Food and IPES-Food, 2017, <www.ipes-food.org>.
6 C. Massy, *Call of the Reed Warbler: A New Agriculture, a New Earth*, University of Queensland Press, Brisbane, 2017.
7 R. Costanza, R. de Groot, P. Sutton, S. van der Ploeg, S. A. Anderson, I. Kubiszewski, S. Farber & R. K. Turner, 'Changes in the Global Value of Ecosystem Services', *Global Environmental Change*, 2014, vol. 26, pp. 152–8.
8 N. Ramankutty, Z. Mehrabi, K. Waha, L. Jarvis, C. Kremen, M. Herrero & L. H. Rieseberg, 'Trends in Global Agricultural Land Use: Implications for Environmental Health and Food Security', *Annual Review of Plant Biology*, 2018, vol. 61, 14.1–14.27.
9 W. Steffen, W. Broadgate, L. Deutsch, O. Gaffney & C. Ludwig, 'The trajectory of the Anthropocene: The Great Acceleration', *The Anthropocene Review*, vol. 2, no. 1, 2015, pp. 81–98.
10 T. Weis, 'The Accelerating Biophysical Contradictions of Industrial Capitalist Agriculture', *Journal of Agrarian Change*, 2010, vol. 10, no. 3, pp. 315–41.
11 IPES-Food, *Too Big to Feed: Exploring the Impacts of Mega-mergers, Consolidation and Concentration of Power in the Agri-food Sector*, 2017, Executive Summary, p. 3 <www.ipes-food.org/images/Reports/Concentration_ExecSummary.pdf>.
12 'Men make their own history, but they do not make it as they please; they do not make it under self-selected circumstances, but under circumstances existing already, given and transmitted from the past.' Karl Marx, *The Eighteenth Brumaire of Louis Bonaparte*, 1852.

NOTES

Appendix – The Urban Agriculture Forum Statement: Urban and Peri-Urban Agriculture Food System Renewal Manifesto

1   'Fast food' is here defined as 'energy-dense, nutrient poor' and predominantly pre-processed and prepared foods in a takeaway/drive-through restaurant: A. M. Prentice & S. A. Jebb, 'Fast Foods, Energy Density and Obesity: A Possible Mechanistic Link', *Obesity Reviews*, 2003, vol. 4, no. 4, pp. 187–94.

Printed in Australia
AUHW011523290719
315228AU00004B/4